Problems in
Gastroenterology

Problems in Practice Series

Problems in Practice Series

Series Editors : J.Fry K.G.D.Williams M.Lancaster-Smith

Problems in Gastroenterology

Michael Lancaster-Smith
BSc,MD,MRCP
Consultant Physician
Queen Mary's Hospital
Sidcup, Kent

Kenneth G.D.Williams
MB,BS,FRCS
Consultant Surgeon
Farnborough Hospital
Orpington, Kent

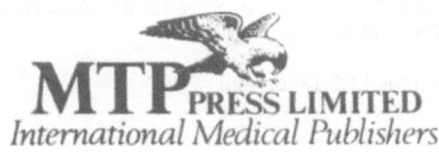
MTP PRESS LIMITED
International Medical Publishers

Published by
MTP Press Limited
Falcon House
Lancaster, England

Copyright © 1982 M. Lancaster-Smith and
Softcover reprint of the hardcover 1st edition 1982
K. G. D. Williams

First published 1982

British Library Cataloguing in Publication Data

Lancaster-Smith, M.
    Problems in gastroenterology.—(Problems in
    practice series)
    1. Gastroenterology
    I. Title   II. Williams, K. G. D.   III. Series
    616.3′3   RC816

ISBN-13: 978-94-011-7208-0   e-ISBN-13: 978-94-011-7206-6
DOI: 10.1007/978-94-011-7206-6

Typesetting by Swiftpages Ltd, Liverpool

Contents

5

Contents

drugs – Alcoholic liver disease – Cirrhosis – Categories
of cirrhosis – Encephalopathy

Preface

Part one of the book presents the gastrointestinal problems that commonly face the general practitioner. Emphasis is placed on analysis of clinical data and how this may provoke the most profitable lines of investigation. Many of the investigation and treatment protocols are within the scope of general practice, but hospital management is also included. It was possible to deal with common oesophageal diseases under the heading of oesophageal problems in Part 1. In contrast, it proved impossible to discuss adequately all of the common diseases affecting other organs of the digestive system under the problem headings. For this reason, a fuller account of many common alimentary diseases is provided in Part two.

M. L.-S.
K. G. D. W.

Series Foreword

This series of books is designed to help general practitioners. So are other books. What is unusual in this instance is their collective authorship; they are written by specialists working at district general hospitals. The writers derive their own experience from a range of cases less highly selected than those on which textbooks are traditionally based. They are also in a good position to pick out topics which they see creating difficulties for the practitioners of their district, whose personal capacities are familiar to them; and to concentrate on contexts where mistakes are most likely to occur. They are all well-accustomed to working in consultation.

All the authors write from hospital experience and from the viewpoint of their specialty. There are, therefore, matters important to family practice which should be sought not within this series, but elsewhere. Within the series much practical and useful advice is to be found with which the general practitioner can compare his existing performance and build in new ideas and improved techniques.

These books are attractively produced and I recommend them.

J. P. Horder CBE
President, The Royal College
of General Practitioners

Part 1
Common Problems

Part I
Common Problems

⓵ Common oesophageal problems

Normal function and structure – Heartburn – Problems with swallowing

Normal function and structure

An understanding of oesophageal function helps to explain some of the common oesophageal problems resulting from dysfunction and leads to a more logical approach to their management.

The primary function of the oesophagus is transport of food and liquid from the pharynx to the stomach. It consists of a tube of muscle lined proximally by squamous epithelium and in the distal few centimetres by columnar cells.

Swallowing   Swallowing is initiated by voluntary contractions of the striated muscle of the pharynx and the upper portion of the oesophagus. The bolus is then propelled to the lower part of the organ by reflex peristaltic action of smooth muscle. The distal 4 centimetres of muscle, though not anatomically distinct, function as a sphincter which relaxes as the peristaltic wave approaches, allowing the bolus to enter the stomach.

Antireflux   The lower oesophageal sphincter (L.O.S.) then rapidly
mechanisms   regains its tone, thus preventing reflux of gastric contents. It is also able to increase its tone still more in response to rises in intragastric and intra-abdominal pressures. The other anti-reflux mechanisms are illustrated in Figure 1.1. The so-called 'pinchcock action' of the diaphragm probably plays only a small part, but the intra-abdominal segment of the oesophagus below the diaphragm which acts as a flap valve is much more important. Any rise in abdominal pressure which raises intra-

15

gastric pressure and encourages reflux will also squeeze equally upon the intra-abdominal oesophagus, thus helping to suppress reflux. Despite these mechanisms most of us intermittently reflux small amounts of gastric fluid. This is rapidly returned to the stomach by reflex muscle action of the distal oesophagus, so-called 'secondary peristalsis'.

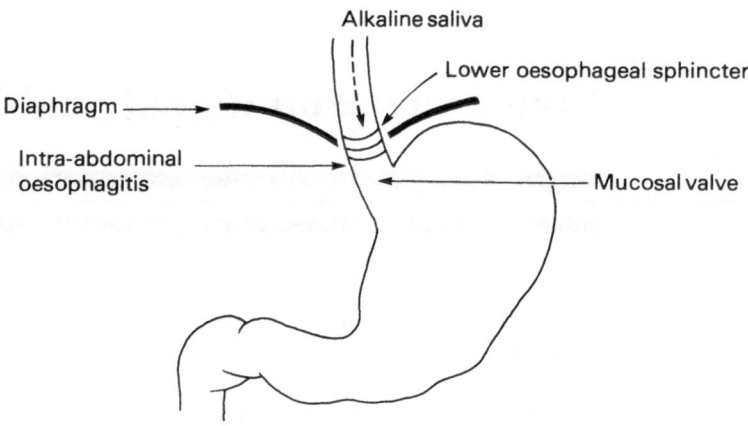

Anti gastro-oesophageal reflux mechanisms

Figure 1.1

Control of muscle activity   The control of this motor activity is not entirely clear, but it is known that an intact myenteric plexus of the oesophageal wall is essential for organized peristalsis. Parasympathetic activity and cholinergic transmitters increase and stimulation by the sympathetic nervous system and adrenergic transmitters decrease tone in the L.O.S. In addition to nervous control, hormones from the upper gastrointestinal tract also affect lower oesophageal function. Although their exact roles are not yet fully understood, gastrin increases L.O.S. tone, whereas secretin has the opposite effect.

Heartburn

The commonest symptom of oesophageal disease is heartburn. This accounts for about 20% of referrals to a district general hospital gastrointestinal clinic.

Gastro-oesophageal reflux   Heartburn is due to irritation of the oesophageal mucosa. This results from excessive contact with noxious gastric contents, as a consequence of continual or recurrent failure of the antireflux mechanisms.

Mechanism of pain

Pain probably arises directly from nerve endings in this hypersensitive mucosa, whenever there is further exposure to irritants such as hydrochloric acid and bile from the stomach or ingested hot drinks and alcoholic spirits. Although in some instances hypersensitivity progresses to frank oesophagitis, inflammatory changes are not present in all patients with heartburn. Why pain arises from the mucosa in the absence of inflammation is not clear, but presumably constant contact with noxious substances renders the mucosa more permeable to irritants and the nerve endings more sensitive. It also seems likely that at least some pain results from spasm in the muscle of the distal oesophagus.

Site

Heartburn, as with other sensations from the oesophagus, is usually felt retrosternally but may also be felt high in the epigastrium and along the costal margins. Radiation to the back of the thorax, neck, shoulders, arms and even the ears is not uncommon.

Nature

As the name implies, patients frequently describe the pain as burning which is felt particularly soon after a meal or whilst swallowing hot liquids or alcoholic spirits. On other occasions the pain will be likened to a lump stuck in the chest or throat. However, this sensation comes on after eating and not whilst eating as in true dysphagia, and there is no actual hold-up of food.

There are a number of other helpful pointers to pain suspected of being due to gastro-oesophageal reflux.

Regurgitation

Posture

Relief

Regurgitation of acid or bitter gastric contents into the mouth frequently occurs. Both regurgitation and heartburn may be brought on by bending or lying down. Antacids or belching often give relief.

When these symptoms occur together there is no diagnostic problem and investigation is unnecessary.

Differential diagnosis

Unfortunately the situation is not always so clear-cut and the diagnosis may have to be distinguished from other oesophageal diseases (see below, dysphagia), peptic ulcer and gallbladder disease (Chapter 4) since similar symptoms may be present.

Confusion with cardiac pain

Because of its site and radiation, heartburn can also be confused with the pain of myocardial ischaemia. However, cardiac pain is usually more severe and described as gripping or crushing and not burning. It is frequently brought on by exertion and not by stooping or lying. There is often accompanying dyspnoea and not belching or regurgitation. The problem can sometimes be further resolved by the therapeutic test of asking the patient

17

to note whether glyceryl trinitrate or antacids give the greater relief.

The continuing diagnostic problem

Nevertheless, there will be a small number in whom the diagnosis is not clear. Both these and those who fail to respond adequately to therapy will require further investigation.

Barium swallow and meal

Barium studies have two main purposes. One is to exclude other disorders of the gastrointestinal tract such as peptic ulcer or carcinoma of the gastric cardia in which reflux symptoms may be prominent. The second is to demonstrate that reflux will

Hiatus hernia

occur and whether there is an accompanying *sliding hiatus hernia*, which predisposes to reflux because the intra-abdominal segment of oesophagus is lost. Nevertheless, it is important to realize that failure to show a hernia does not exclude the diagnosis of gastro-oesophageal reflux as this can certainly exist in those without a hiatus hernia. It should also be stressed that a hernia itself does not cause symptoms unless accompanied by reflux. Likewise, some patients only have intermittent reflux and the radiologist may not be able to confirm its presence despite using various manoeuvres to stress the anti-reflux mechanisms.

Endoscopy

Examination of the oesophagus, stomach and proximal duodenum with a flexible fibre optic instrument is a safe and well tolerated outpatient procedure now available in most district general hospitals. The patient is sedated with intravenous diazepam and the pharynx anaesthetized with benzo-caine or xylocaine. The examination lasts approximately 10 minutes and the patient can return home within 2 hours, provided he is accompanied. Because of residual drowsiness he should not drive for the remainder of the day.

Oesophagitis

Obvious inflammatory changes of oesophagitis, assessed either by direct vision or histologically, may not always be present even in patients with severe heartburn. Thus, to some extent endoscopy has proved disappointing in the investigation of gastro-oesophageal reflux. Nevertheless, it may be helpful when diagnosis or management is proving difficult, and is obligatory if in addition to heartburn there is dysphagia, anorexia, weight loss or vomiting.

Acid perfusion

(Bernstein test)

If there is still doubt about the diagnosis of heartburn, its precipitation by the perfusion into the distal oesophagus of N/10 hydrochloric acid and subsequent relief with sodium bicarb-onate may be helpful.

18

Manometry
and pH
recording

In rare cases more information about the exact nature of the reflux problem can occasionally be of use. This can be obtained by intraluminal pressure measurements which assess lower oesophageal muscle dysfunction and by intraluminal pH probes which accurately and objectively record the frequency of reflux episodes. Such procedures are only indicated when the other simpler and more readily available techniques have failed to confirm the diagnosis.

Management

The management of most cases of heartburn poses few problems.

Improve
L.O.S. function

The first aim is to *improve the efficiency of the antireflux mechanisms and reduce the demands made upon them.* Certain foods, particularly fats, regularly cause heartburn and probably do so by changing the levels of the hormones that control L.O.S. tone. The patient has usually discovered this for himself and taken the necessary action. Alcohol and smoking both reduce the efficiency of the L.O.S. and should be avoided, especially at meal times. Metoclopramide (Maxolon and Primperan), as it improves L.O.S. function and enhances secondary peristalsis, is worthy of trial. It should be taken prior to meals and before going to bed.

Reduction of
intragastric
pressure

Warning should be given not to take large meals and large volumes of fluid or to drink with a meal, as this may increase intragastric pressure to a level that overcomes the antireflux mechanisms. This is most likely to happen when the meal is followed by lying down, slumping in a chair or stooping. Specific advice must therefore be given about posture, even to the extent of raising the head of the bed by about 10 cm or elevating the mattress with pillows beneath the head end.

Weight
reduction

Reduction of weight is a great help when the patient is overweight, even if only a few kilograms are shed. This results in a lowering of intra-abdominal pressure, but the benefit is probably as much due to the accompanying reduction in size of meals.

Alkalis

Pain from a hypersensitive or inflamed mucosa will be decreased by *making gastric contents less acidic.* This can be achieved by regular therapy over a period of a few weeks rather than just when symptoms arise. Taken at this frequency it is probably best to use a combined aluminium and magnesium preparation to avoid bowel disturbance.

Antacids, in addition to their local intraluminal action, tend to reduce reflux itself because alkalinization of the stomach contents stimulates release of gastrin and possibly other hormones which increases L.O.S. tone.

H$_2$ antagonists   The H$_2$ antagonist cimetidine (Tagamet) by suppressing gastric acid secretion will similarly reduce acidity, but because of cost *should be reserved for those cases in which treatment with antacids is unsuccessful.*

Siloxanes and alginates   Preparations combining antacids with polysiloxanes (Asilone, Andursil, Polycrol) are said to form a protective layer and by dispersing intragastric gases reduce belching and reflux. Alginates (Gaviscon, Gastrocote) form an alkaline 'raft' on the gastric contents which suppresses reflux and prevents contact of the gastric fluid and oesophageal mucosa.

Carbenoxylone   Liquorice extracts enhance healing of gastric and duodenal ulcers and their action depends upon contact with the mucosal surface (see Chapter 15, Peptic ulcer). A new product, Pyrogastrone, which combines alginate and carbenoxylone, is intended to deliver the active substance to the inflamed oesophageal mucosa and promote healing.

It should again be stressed that regular antacids prove successful in the great majority of patients with heartburn and other products are only necessary when these have failed.

Avoid anticholinergics   Drugs such as atropine, hyoscine, belladonna and synthetic 'antispasmodics' reduce tone in the L.O.S. and are, therefore, contraindicated in heartburn.

Reassurance   Because of the common association of retrosternal pain with cardiac ischaemia many patients suspect that their pain arises from the heart. Strong reassurance that this is not the case is often required and such reassurance, together with the treatment already discussed, is usually sufficient to abolish or reduce symptoms to a tolerable level.

Special problems

Apart from hiatus hernia and obesity, which have already been mentioned, there are two other common situations which predispose to gastro-oesophageal reflux, i.e. pregnancy and gastric surgery.

Pregnancy   Pregnancy is often accompanied by heartburn and is probably encouraged by a rise in intra-abdominal pressure and a reduction in the tone of the L.O.S.

Gastric surgery   Patients who have undergone gastric surgery, including vagotomy, are prone to heartburn. This is partly caused by irritant bile salts which frequently reflux into the stomach

20

following such operations. Aluminium hydroxide or hydrotalcite (Altacite), both of which bind bile salts, should therefore, be taken regularly until symptoms are relieved.

Scleroderma
A fortunately much rarer condition that also predisposes to gastro-oesophageal reflux is scleroderma. This is because involvement of the oesophageal muscle leads to impaired peristalsis and inefficient clearing of the gullet. The lower oesophageal sphincter is also commonly affected, which allows free flow of gastric contents into the oesophagus. In addition to the symptoms of heartburn and regurgitation, true dysphagia can occur either from impaired peristalsis or from peptic stricture. All that can be offered are those measures prescribed for other severe cases of gastro-oesophageal reflux.

Surgery
Only a very small number of patients with heartburn will require surgery and in these cases there is frequently a substantial coexisting hiatus hernia. The operations with the greatest chance of success aim to reduce the hernia and establish an intra-abdominal segment of oesophagus. The indications for referral to the surgeon are as follows.

(1) Failure of enthusiastic and compliant medical treatment to relieve symptoms or heal oesophagitis.

Haemorrhage
(2) Recurrent haemorrhage either from oesophagitis or an actual oesophageal ulcer – this may present as haematemesis or melaena requiring admission to hospital. However, it is usually occult and *all patients with recurrent heartburn should have a haemoglobin estimation as chronic blood loss and anaemia frequently go undetected both by patient and doctor.*

(3) Stricture, which results from chronic oesophagitis and leads to dysphagia (see below).

Problems with swallowing

The term *dysphagia* should be reserved for difficulty in the act of swallowing. In this situation the bolus will not pass from mouth to stomach or does so only after delay. The problem is often, but not always, accompanied by pain which has the same distribution as that described in the section on heartburn.

False dysphagia

With a carefully taken history this true dysphagia can usually be distinguished from so-called 'false dysphagia'.

21

Gastro-
oesophageal
reflux

As already mentioned, when discussing heartburn, patients with gastro-oesophageal reflux frequently complain of a feeling that there is a lump of food stuck in the chest or throat. In contrast to true dysphagia this sensation *follows* meals, does not occur when actually swallowing and is frequently relieved by antacids.

Cortical
inhibition

Another form of false dysphagia, which is not clearly understood, is found in old age and in the mentally disturbed. The main complaint is that despite masticating food for long periods there is a fear that it will not be successfully swallowed. Such patients therefore fail to pass the food from mouth to pharynx and the bolus is eventually spat out. Tablets often cause a similar problem. Fluids, on the other hand, are swallowed with ease and this can be a useful test in distinguishing the problem from other forms of dysphagia. If the condition is persistent, drugs and nutrition should be given in liquid form. The fundamental disturbance is presumably at cortical level but the exact mechanism is unknown.

Globus
hystericus

Another symptom that is sometimes confused with true dysphagia is the sensation of a lump in the throat which cannot be cleared. It is not related to the act of swallowing or to meals. The term 'globus hystericus' is often applied to this condition, but it is probably best reserved for those patients in whom the symptom is accompanied by firm evidence of psychiatric disturbance. The symptom should always be taken seriously, and if persistent it is advisable to arrange examination of the larynx and pharynx. This will exclude an organic lesion and if negative the reassurance given to the patient will be valuable therapy.

The questions that must be asked in order to distinguish between true and false dysphagia are: 'Does food actually stick during the act of swallowing?' or 'Is there just a sensation of a lump in the throat or chest, which is only present after swallowing, or has no relationship to eating and drinking whatsoever?'

True dysphagia

Pharyngeal
dysphagia

Types of true dysphagia are now considered. If dysphagia occurs almost immediately after attempting to initiate a swallow, the lesion is likely to be in the pharynx. The common causes of this type of dysphagia are:

(1) Pharyngeal pouch
(2) Pharyngo-oesophageal web

22

Common oesophageal problems

(3) Post-cricoid carcinoma
(4) Neuromuscular diseases.

Pharyngeal pouch

The characteristic pattern of symptoms in this condition is discomfort in the throat which occurs rapidly after starting to swallow. This is accompanied by a portion of the bolus returning to the mouth. It usually occurs within a few seconds although on some occasions it may not happen until several hours later. Frequently the patient will have noticed that changes in the position of the head and neck, palpation over one side of the neck or lying down causes a return of food to the mouth. This is often associated with coughing due to aspiration into the respiratory tract. A barium swallow will confirm the diagnosis, but it is important to inform the radiologist that a pouch is suspected, so that special attention is given to examining the early stages of the swallow.

The aetiology and pathogenesis of these pouches is not clear, but it seems likely that there is incoordination of pharyngeal muscle activity at the initiation of swallowing which generates excessive pressure in the pharynx. This results in herniation of the mucous membrane between the inferior constrictor and cricopharyngeus muscles.

Most patients require only explanation of their symptoms and reassurance. However, surgical repair will be needed for those in whom large quantities collect in the diverticulum, especially if there is aspiration into the lungs.

Pharyngo-oesophageal web or stricture

Obstruction of *solid food* at the start of swallowing, in the absence of any difficulty with liquids, is typical of a pharyngo-oesophageal web. As the condition progresses, usually over a period of years, swallowing of liquids also becomes slower and its turbulent flow audible. In severe cases even fluid may be rejected and choking is then common. The lesion takes the form of either a web of mucosa or a smooth intramural annular stricture. The aetiology is not known, but in some cases there is an associated iron deficiency anaemia as initially described by Patterson and Kelley and Plummer and Vinson. It is possible that iron deficiency predisposes the upper alimentary tract to mechanical and thermal trauma, but it is not the total explanation as the same lesions also frequently occur in patients without iron deficiency.

The radiologist will be able to confirm the diagnosis, providing an adequate examination of the upper oesophagus is made. All patients should be referred to a throat specialist for oesophagoscopy and resection of the web or dilatation of the stricture. If there is accompanying iron deficiency the cause

23

should be sought and treated, together with replenishment of iron stores. Recurrence of dysphagia is common because the lesion tends to re-form. It should also be remembered that this condition may be complicated subsequently by post-cricoid carcinoma.

Post-cricoid carcinoma
Symptoms similar to those of pharyngo-oesophageal web, but more rapidly progressive over months rather than years, are suggestive of post-cricoid cancer. In addition, there is often an accompanying continuous discomfort in the throat which is impossible to clear. Early referral to a laryngologist for endoscopic examination is vital. Surgery combined with radiotherapy frequently leads to cure.

Neuro-muscular disease
Failure to shut off the nose and larynx from the pharynx at the start of swallowing, because of neuromuscular dysfunction, leads to food and especially liquids spilling into the nasal passages and lower respiratory tract. When asked to drink the patient will immediately start to cough and splutter. Spillage into the lungs may eventually lead to aspiration pneumonia and lung abscess. Distinction from mechanical obstruction is not a problem as there are usually other neuromuscular symptoms and signs, particularly dysarthria. The commonest conditions giving rise to neuromuscular dysphagia are motor neuron disease, disseminated sclerosis, recurrent strokes and muscular dystrophies. Advanced Parkinsonism may also impair transfer of food from mouth to pharynx because of rigidity and tremor of the tongue.

Many patients can manage solids and thick purées and only have difficulty with liquids and saliva. If adequate nutrition cannot be maintained in a patient whose quality of life is otherwise satisfactory, a thin, highly flexible nasogastric tube can be used to give a balanced liquid diet. If there is sufficient support this treatment can continue on a long term basis at home.

Oesophageal dysphagia
Dysphagia caused by oesophageal disease or cancer of the gastric fundus is readily distinguished from pharyngeal dysphagia because in the former there is a delay between starting to swallow and the sensation of obstruction. The common causes of this type of dysphagia are benign and carcinomatous oesophageal stricture, achalasia and carcinoma of the gastric fundus.

Oesophageal stricture

The vast majority of oesophageal strictures are due either to carcinoma or to peptic oesophagitis. A few are the result of

24

Distinction between benign and malignant strictures swallowed corrosives. Distinction between cancer and benign peptic stricture can frequently be made from the clinical findings. Patients with benign peptic lesions, because they are caused by gastro-oesophageal reflux and resulting oesophagitis, often give a history of previous heartburn and pain induced by alcohol and hot liquids. In contrast, a preceding history of pain is rare when malignancy is the cause. With benign strictures the tendency for solids to obstruct is often initially intermittent and increases in severity over a period of months, whereas carcinoma leads to rapidly progressive dysphagia with a total history of only a few weeks. Despite their longstanding symptoms patients with benign stricture present with a comparatively normal state of nutrition and a well preserved appetite. In contrast, those with carcinoma have usually lost weight; this is due as much to anorexia as the dysphagia itself. In patients with peptic stricture, liquids may continue to pass without undue trouble almost indefinitely, but cancer will eventually lead to complete blockage.

When a bolus of food impacts in the narrowed segment, whether the lesion is malignant or benign, the patient will find it necessary *to induce regurgitation* in order to clear the obstruction and ease pain. This differs from the spontaneous regurgitation of gastric fluid which occurs in patients with uncomplicated gastro-oesophageal reflux.

Fibre optic endoscopy and radiology are essential investigations for the patient suffering from this group of symptoms.

Radiology Benign strictures appear on barium swallow in one of two forms. The more common are circumferential with smoothly tapering sides. They are usually less than 2 cm in length and tend to occur at the junction of the squamous and columnar epithelium. Less frequently the benign stricture appears as a short, smooth-walled cuff, but also involving the whole circumference of the distal oesophagus. This is the so-called 'Schatzski's ring' and consists of fibrous tissue extending from the submucosal layers to the serosa. The epithelium has a normal appearance. Such lesions are considered to be the result of oesophagitis, but why the epithelium itself is not overtly involved remains unclear. Unlike peptic strictures, which are virtually restricted to the distal oesophagus, carcinoma may occur at any site. Malignant strictures are longer than benign lesions, usually greater than 2 cm, and the profile on barium swallow is often asymmetrical.

Endoscopy Fibre optic endoscopy is complementary to radiology and should be performed early. It makes possible a direct assessment of the nature and extent of the lesion. Furthermore, because it provides a means of obtaining biopsies and material for cytology, an accurate tissue diagnosis can be made in the majority of patients. This will assist in deciding about the course **Management** of future management, which is clearly dependent upon whether the stricture is benign or malignant. Whilst awaiting a definitive diagnosis the patient should be advised to eat no solids and maintain nutrition by taking fortified milk and soups. This will prevent complete obstruction and collection of debris in the oesophagus, thus facilitating endoscopic examination.

Oesophageal carcinoma

About 75% of oesophageal cancers are squamous cell lesions and 25% are adenocarcinomas. The latter occur in the distal third and arise from gastric mucosa that has extended into the lower oesophagus. The greatest incidence of oesophageal carcinoma is in the over-60 age group. Those in the lower two thirds are twice as common in males as females, but post-cricoid tumours occur more frequently in women than men. Aetiological factors include heavy smoking, excessive alcohol and, as already mentioned, post-cricoid cancer can complicate the Patterson–Kelley syndrome. Achalasia is also associated with an increased incidence of carcinoma and is presumably due to prolonged contact of the mucosa with carcinogens from stagnating food in the aperistaltic oesophagus.

The prognosis is poor, with an overall 5-year survival of approximately 10%. Treatment is by surgery or radiotherapy, but the relative merits of each are still undecided. Surgery is attempted for tumours involving the distal two thirds. In operable cases the surgeon is usually able to obtain clearance of the lesion yet still able to join the proximal oesophagus to stomach. In some patients this is not possible and a segment of colon has to be transplanted in order to provide continuity. It is claimed that radiotherapy gives results equal to those of surgery in cancers of the upper third of the oesophagus. Some centres have adopted a combined therapeutic approach but the results do not appear to be dramatically different from surgery alone.

When cure is impossible, usually because of local spread within the mediastinum, radiotherapy often proves of value as a palliative measure, temporarily relieving dysphagia and blood loss. An alternative palliative procedure for dysphagia is the insertion of a Mousseau Barbin or Celestin tube. These are wide-bore tubes than can be passed orally down the oesophagus and through the stricture into the stomach. In the past, positioning of the tube has necessitated a gastrotomy, but it can now be inserted without this operation by using special apparatus in conjunction with a fibre optic endoscope. The tube permits a liquid diet which can maintain adequate nutrition for several months. Unfortunately, it is not without its own complications which include aspiration pneumonitis, blockage with food and tumour or erosion and perforation into the mediastinum.

Benign peptic stricture

Peptic stricture is caused by subepithelial fibrosis. This is the consequence of an inflammatory reaction resulting from refluxed gastric acid and bile. It is usually, though not invariably, preceded by a long history of gastro-oesophageal reflux symptoms. The condition, having been confirmed, and distinguished from cancer by endoscopy, is best managed in the majority of cases by dilatation. The use of endoscopically positioned Eder Peustow dilators has made this a safe and convenient treatment. The patient requires admission for only 24 h. The number of dilations before achieving full patency of the oesophagus varies considerably. However, when patency has been established, recurrence of the stricture can usually be prevented by enthusiastic medical management of the underlying gastro-oesophageal reflux. In those patients where there is rapid and frequent recurrence, particularly if young, referral for resection of the stricture and antireflux surgery should be seriously considered.

Achalasia

Compared with benign peptic stricture and carcinoma of the oesophagus, achalasia is a relatively rare cause of dysphagia. It can usually be distinguished from the former two conditions by careful attention to the clinical features.

For several years before presentation many patients have experienced *spontaneous* central chest pain. It is often severe and has the same distribution as pain from gastro-oesophageal reflux. In contrast, there is no definite relationship to food and because of the severity and 'bursting' nature of the pain there may be confusion with cardiac ischaemia. At this stage some patients also will have noticed intermittent dysphagia, although many have no trouble with swallowing until several years later. In contrast to dysphagia due to stricture, fluids, even from the beginning, give as much trouble as solids. Achalasia may cause remarkably little incapacity because the patient frequently learns that by his *eating small quantities slowly* the oesophagus will accept moderate quantities of food. Eventually the lower oesophageal sphincter is forced open and the food enters the stomach. If a meal is taken too quickly the capacity of the oesophagus to accommodate food is overcome, which results in regurgitation. Unlike that associated with gastro-oesophageal reflux, the regurgitated matter tastes only of the swallowed food and not of bile or acid. Sometimes regurgitation only occurs when the patient is recumbent, which leads to explosive nocturnal coughing and occasionally to aspiration pneumonitis.

Swallowed air cannot enter the stomach in achalasia, which results in the absence of a gastric fundal air bubble on chest X-ray. This is sometimes a useful chance finding in patients who have been referred for chest X-ray because their predominant symptom is chest pain.

Radiology

As in all cases of true dysphagia, an early barium swallow is required. This will show absent or reduced peristalsis of the oesophagus and non-relaxation of the lower oesophageal sphincter. By the time most patients are investigated, the oesophagus will have dilated and developed an 'S' shaped configuration. Unlike the narrowed segment in carcinoma, which is long and irregular, in achalasia the segment is smooth and tapering.

Endoscopy

Endoscopy will confirm the diagnosis and will completely exclude peptic or carcinomatous stricture. An inflamed and oedematous mucosa is often seen, which is caused by irritation from stagnant food.

Pathology and aetiology

The underlying pathological lesion is absence or reduction of the ganglionic cells in Auerbach's plexus. Dysphagia results from a combination of absent or inadequate peristalsis and failure of the lower oesophageal sphincter to relax. The cause is unknown but, because lymphocytic infiltration is found in many cases, a viral or autoimmune aetiology has been proposed.

Treatment

There is *no* satisfactory drug therapy and referral for surgery is advisable as soon as the degree of dysphagia becomes unacceptable to the patient. Recurrent aspiration into the respiratory tract is a further indication for surgery.

Cardiomyotomy

The operation of choice is cardiomyotomy (Heller's operation), which consists of cutting the muscle layers of the distal oesophagus down to the mucosa. Results are usually satisfactory but dysphagia may persist if the surgeon is too conservative. Because the operation disrupts the lower oesophageal sphincter, reflux of gastric contents commonly occurs and may

Dilatation

Complications

itself become a clinical problem in some patients.

The only alternative treatment to Heller's operation is dilatation of the lower oesophageal sphincter with inflatable bougies under radiological control. The procedure often has to be repeated and the overall results are not as satisfactory as those achieved by myotomy.

Aspiration has already been discussed.

Bleeding from the congested and inflamed mucosa may cause anaemia or, more rarely, haematemesis and melaena.

A more serious problem is the undoubted increased incidence of *carcinoma of the oesophagus*. Presentation is late and prognosis extremely poor. The clinician should be alerted to the possibility of a malignancy by worsening dysphagia, anaemia, anorexia and weight loss. Unfortunately, there is little evidence that Heller's operation reduces the risk of developing cancer. As yet there is no information about the value of long term endoscopically monitored follow-up for the 'early' detection of malignancy.

Other disorders that cause dysphagia

The great majority of all patients with oesophageal dysphagia will be found to have peptic or carcinomatous stricture or achalasia.

Nevertheless, a number of other conditions may lead to dysphagia, although it is rarely the presenting or predominant symptom in these disorders. Such conditions include *scleroderma* and *dermatomyositis*, both of which are usually obvious from other characteristic features of the disease. *Carcinoma of the bronchus* or *lymphoma* involving mediastinal nodes may sometimes cause dysphagia either by invasion or extrinsic pressure. Other signs are usually present and chest X-ray will clarify the situation. Pain whilst swallowing may also be caused by *candidiasis* of the oesophagus. The characteristic white lesions are also frequently present in the mouth and pharynx. It is most commonly found in diabetics and those taking steroids, antibiotics or cytotoxic drugs. It should be treated with nystatin or amphotericin B.

Conclusion

In summary, when confronted with a patient who complains of a problem with swallowing, the first task is to decide whether this is true dysphagia or does the patient really have one of the

29

conditions mentioned in the section on false dysphagia. This distinction is important because, as discussed, the investigations and management are quite different. Careful listening and questioning will separate the true dysphagias into pharyngeal and oesophageal causes. *A short history, accompanied by anorexia and weight loss, points towards cancer.* True dysphagia must also be distinguished from the 'sensation of a lump' that occurs in many patients with uncomplicated gastro-oesophageal reflux. In this latter condition there is no obstruction of the bolus and the sensation comes on after and not during the swallow. Early radiology and endoscopy are indicated in all cases of true dysphagia except those with obvious neuromuscular disease of the pharynx. In contrast, those patients with uncomplicated gastro-oesophageal reflux do not require immediate investigation. They should be treated initially along the lines already discussed in the section on heartburn, and investigation should only be undertaken if the problem persists.

Points to stress

Distinction between benign and malignant oesophageal strictures

Benign	Malignant
Previous heartburn common	Previous pain uncommon
Often intermittent dysphagia for many months	Progressive dysphagia for a few weeks
Weight and appetite maintained	Weight loss and anorexia

Investigations and therapy

- The great majority of patients with uncomplicated gastro-oesophageal reflux will respond to adequate antacid therapy and where appropriate, weight reduction.
- When these measures fail other preparations, such as cimetidine, metoclopramide, pyrogastrone, Gaviscon or Gastrocote should be tried.
- Check haemoglobin concentration as anaemia may go unnoticed.
- Other investigations are only necessary when diagnosis is unclear or when there is accompanying *dysphagia* or *anorexia.*
- The demonstration of an hiatus hernia is not essential for the diagnosis of gastro-oesophageal reflux.

Common oesophageal problems

The sensation of a lump stuck in the chest or throat

- Soon after eating a meal – gastro-oesophageal reflux.
- Whilst swallowing – stricture (peptic or carcinoma).
- Not related to eating – globus syndrome or laryngeal disease.

Factors which increase the chance of gastro-oesophageal reflux

- Raised intragastric pressure (large meals and volumes of liquid).
- Lying and stooping.
- Obesity.
- Pregnancy.
- Gastric surgery.
- Alcohol and smoking.
- Scleroderma.
- Hiatus hernia with loss of intra-abdominal oesophagus.

2 Nausea and vomiting

Patients complaining of nausea and vomiting can usually be placed in one of three categories – acute, persistent or episodic. In most situations, nausea and vomiting are closely associated. The former is usually a premonitory symptom to the act of vomiting, though it frequently occurs alone. In contrast, vomiting in the absence of nausea is rare.

Acute vomiting

Acute vomiting or a single brief episode of vomiting may accompany many disorders. They are invariably accompanied or rapidly followed by other symptoms or signs, which facilitate diagnosis. Thus, the diarrhoea and malaise that accompany vomiting, caused by *viral and bacterial infection* of the gastro-intestinal tract, usually makes the diagnosis obvious. Profound anorexia and nausea more often than vomiting are typical of *viral hepatitis*, often preceding jaundice by several days. The onset of *biliary colic and pancreatitis* is sometimes accompanied by vomiting, the mechanism of which is not clear. It might be a non-specific response to pain because many painful conditions, such as *myocardial infarction* and *renal colic*, sometimes result in vomiting. In these latter disorders vomiting may confuse the situation, diverting attention away from the underlying problem.

Acute vestibulitis and vascular disease involving the cerebellar connections give rise to severe vertigo and frequently vomiting. *Raised intracranial pressure* resulting from *malignant hypertension* or *intracranial tumour* and *haemorrhage* are well recognized causes of vomiting. Preceding nausea is said not to occur.

33

Persistent vomiting

In these conditions vomiting is often prominent, though rarely the only symptom. Thus, diagnosis is not usually a problem. Successful management usually depends upon correction of the underlying condition.

Gastro-intestinal diseases *Pyloric stenosis,* due to either carcinoma of the stomach or chronic duodenal ulcer, gives rise to persistent large-volume vomiting. Food eaten many hours previously can be identified and a succussion splash is often produced by vigorous palpation of the upper abdomen. Vomiting is a feature of *intestinal obstruction.* It is characteristically accompanied by colic and abdominal distension. Pyloric stenosis and intestinal obstruction require urgent admission to hospital for correction of electrolyte imbalance and gastric aspiration. Surgical intervention is usually necessary in both conditions.

Non-gastro-intestinal disease A large number of women in early *pregnancy* suffer from nausea and vomiting. It tends to be most severe on rising each morning. Only rarely does the condition lead to dehydration and in the majority resolves completely by the end of the first trimester. Some patients omit to mention or deny the possibility of pregnancy. In such cases examination of the breasts for signs of pregnancy and a history of amenorrhoea will avoid unnecessary investigation.

Almost any *drug* should be suspected as a potential cause of vomiting and nausea, particularly if recently prescribed. Anti-inflammatory analgesics, cytotoxics and some antibiotics are frequently to blame. Morphine, codeine and their derivatives commonly induce nausea and vomiting. Digoxin should also be remembered as a cause of these symptoms, especially in the elderly and those with renal impairment.

Vomiting may be a prominent symptom in *endocrine* and *metabolic disease.* Vomiting in association with constipation, muscle weakness and depression should raise the suspicion of *hypercalcaemia. Addison's disease* commonly and *thyrotoxicosis,* less frequently, present with unexplained vomiting. The underlying cause in Addison's disease is thought to be hyponatraemia because patients with *sodium deficiency* from other disorders also suffer from severe nausea and vomiting. *Hepatic and renal failure* of any aetiology are frequently complicated by persistent vomiting.

Episodic vomiting

There are many conditions of diverse aetiology that give rise to episodic vomiting. Because in many instances the attacks are brief and resolve spontaneously, several episodes may occur before the patient seeks medical advice.

Psychogenic
vomiting

Psychological disturbance is by far the commonest cause of periodic nausea and vomiting, especially when these symptoms occur in apparent isolation. In susceptible individuals vomiting may be precipitated by acute stress. In more prolonged stressful situations or when there is unresolved conflict, vomiting may become a chronic or recurrent problem. If the doctor, patient or relatives are able to identify these factors the diagnosis is not difficult. Because a history of stress or conflict is not always forthcoming from the patient, it is usually necessary to interview relatives and friends. Features of organic disease are absent and only rarely is there significant weight loss or electrolyte disturbance. Accompanying anxiety and depression are often alleviated by the onset of vomiting. This can be explained partly by increased sympathy and attention from relatives and friends following the development of a more readily understandable physical symptom. It is not uncommon for alimentary psychogenic symptoms to occur in patients who have suffered previously from organic gastrointestinal disease. It is particularly important to rule out recurrence of the old problem in such patients. In children and infants, cyclical vomiting is frequently the result of emotional disturbance due to domestic tensions. In children, unhappy at school, vomiting may allow them to stay at home. A very small number of women suffer from brief bouts of vomiting at a particular time in their menstrual cycle. Whether it has a hormonal or psychological cause is not known.

The crucial factor in management of psychogenic vomiting is identification and removal of the underlying problem. Antidepressants and tranquillizers may also be useful when depression and anxiety are prominent.

Anorexia
nervosa

A quite separate group of psychologically disturbed patients who often present with episodic vomiting are those suffering from anorexia nervosa. The overwhelming number are female, between 15 and 30 years of age. Diagnosis depends upon eliciting the other typical features of the disease from both patient and relatives. These include weight loss, avoidance of dietary carbohydrate, amenorrhoea, overactivity and the patient's distorted impression of her body size and image. In addition to the vomiting, which may be spontaneous or induced, many also resort to laxative and diuretic abuse (p. 93). Management is difficult and success depends upon altering the attitude towards food and body image. A commonly adopted policy is to

35

get the patient to increase her daily calories gradually, in exchange for simple rewards. The setting of weight targets for specific deadlines is also important. When present, depression and psychoses must also be treated.

Alcohol

Vomiting and retching on first rising are common symptoms of alcohol abuse. Curiously, patients either fail to realize, or refuse to admit, that alcohol could be the cause of the problem. This may delay the diagnosis and lead to unnecessary investigation. All patients suffering from this symptom must, therefore, be specifically questioned about alcohol consumption. A positive history is not always forthcoming. Friends and relatives should then be interviewed before investigating the alimentary tract. Pressure to arrange gastrointestinal studies is often increased by coexistent diarrhoea. This, however, can also be caused by excessive alcohol. Positive proof that alcohol is to blame often depends upon resolution of vomiting after admission to hospital and enforced abstinence. The finding of a high mean red cell volume or serum γ-glutamyltransferase supports this diagnosis. The mechanism is not clear but seems likely to be as much due to central nervous system disturbance as gastric irritation.

Migraine

Nausea and vomiting may form a prominent feature of migraine. The characteristic headache and prodromal symptoms, such as teichopsia and hemianopia, usually make the diagnosis obvious. A minority of patients also experience abdominal pain during an attack of migraine, which may cause confusion and stimulate a search for gastrointestinal disease.

Meniere's and cerebellar disease

When vertigo occurs in Meniere's disease and disseminated sclerosis it is often accompanied by vomiting. Other vestibular or neurological symptoms and signs are usually present.

Peptic disease

Recurrent vomiting in the absence of pain is very rare in peptic ulcer. Gastro-oesophageal reflux, leading to regurgitation of stomach contents into the mouth, sometimes induces vomiting, which is not preceded or accompanied by nausea. A careful history will elicit the true sequence of events. Vomiting of gastric contents, which often contain large amounts of bile, occurs in a small but significant number of patients who have undergone *partial gastrectomy*. It tends to decrease with time and only rarely warrants further surgery.

Points to stress

Episodic vomiting

• *Psychogenic causes are commonest.*

- *Vomiting with amenorrhoea and weight loss in adolescence – consider anorexia nervosa.*
- *Vomiting soon after waking in the morning is usually due to alcohol abuse.*
- *Vomiting without abdominal pain is rarely due to peptic ulcer.*

③ The acute abdomen

Many excellent and traditional textbooks of surgery have been written on the principles of diagnosis of acute abdominal disease. It is, therefore, not intended to repeat information which can be easily obtained elsewhere. This chapter is not intended as a comprehensive guide to the acute abdomen, but emphasizes the diagnostic features and management of commonly occurring diseases.

The admitting diagnoses on patients entering a busy surgical ward will be as follows:

(1) *Inflammatory disease* – (a) appendicitis, (b) gallbladder disease, (c) diverticular disease, (d) pancreatitis.

(2) *Obstructive causes* – small bowel obstruction, large bowel obstruction.

(3) *Perforation* – stomach, duodenum, large and small bowel.

(4) *Gynaecological problems* – pelvic inflammatory disease, ectopic pregnancy.

(5) *Less common diagnoses* – aortic aneurysm, ischaemic bowel disease.

Diagnosis   Successful management of the acute abdomen is directly related to the early diagnosis and institution of correct treatment. A thorough history and careful physical examination will produce an accurate or working diagnosis in the majority of patients.

39

Inflammatory disease

Appendicitis

Appendicitis is the commonest cause of pain in the right iliac fossa. It is no respecter of age, but most commonly occurs in patients below the age of 25. Classical symptoms include central abdominal pain moving to the right iliac fossa, anorexia and a mild pyrexia. Tenderness and guarding present at an early stage. The diagnosis is essentially made by palpation of the right iliac fossa. Two common conditions which are often impossible to differentiate from appendicitis are mesenteric adenitis and right-sided salpingitis. It may be necessary to examine the patient several times over a period of hours before a definite diagnosis can be made. If there is any doubt it is wiser to perform an appendicectomy and inspect the pelvic organs at the same time.

Problems in diagnosis

Problems in diagnosis are the retrocaecal appendix, mesenteric adenitis, appendicitis in obese patients, pelvic appendicitis and appendicitis in pregnancy.

Retrocaecal appendix

With the retrocaecal appendix, the signs of appendicitis may be masked owing to the overlying caecum. As the inflammation increases, it induces an ileus in the caecum and this in itself makes palpation of the appendix difficult. Often peritoneal irritation occurs late in these patients. It is not uncommon to find that the patient has been generally unwell for 24–48 h before complaining of a significant abdominal pain.

Mesenteric adenitis

Mesenteric adenitis is usually associated with children below the age of 12, although over the past few years epidemics of a similar condition have occurred in young adults. The patient complains of vague lower abdominal pain mainly in the right iliac fossa, associated with loss of appetite. There is often a previous history of an upper respiratory tract or throat infection. The patient may appear flushed and has lower abdominal guarding, more so in the right iliac fossa. Bowel sounds are often hyperactive. Temperature is often elevated. The white count may show a leukocytosis. If the diagnosis is correct, a general improvement in the patient's condition will appear within 24 h. If there is any doubt it is wiser to remove the appendix. Needless to say, many normal appendices are removed because of this difficulty in diagnosis.

Appendicitis in pregnancy

In the early stages of pregnancy the appendix is to be found within the right iliac fossa. As the uterus enlarges, the appendix rises in the abdomen and may eventually lie in the right hypochondrium. Therefore, in pregnancy the signs and symptoms remain the same but the site changes.

Pelvic appendix

A very small proportion of patients have an appendix which is long and in the pelvic position, i.e. it lies across the pelvic brim and extends into the true pelvis itself. It has been suggested that the inflamed appendix may be felt rectally. The author's own experience is that in those patients who have tenderness rectally also have obvious signs of appendicitis on abdominal examination. Rectal examination appears to be useful in differentiating salpingitis from appendicitis, but is of little value in making the diagnosis of appendicitis.

Obesity

Beware of the obese patient with pain in the right iliac fossa. Often the thickness of the fat in the right iliac fossa will make adequate palpation unsatisfactory; it is wise to admit obese patients with suspected appendicitis to hospital immediately. It is in this group of patients that the white blood count is a useful investigation.

Management of appendicitis

Immediate appendicectomy is the only satisfactory treatment for appendicitis. Medical management is contraindicated except in unusual circumstances, i.e. on board ship, mountaineering etc. Antibiotics have no place in the treatment of appendicitis, and the practice of giving antibiotics indiscriminately to children with lower abdominal pain should be condemned.

Appendix mass

An appendix mass is produced by the localization of the inflamed – often gangrenous – appendix by the omentum. The omentum itself contributes to the greater size of the mass.

Management of appendix mass

The majority of appendix masses slowly decreases in size with conservative treatment. However, if the mass increases in size or there are signs of septicaemia or spreading peritonitis, the underlying abscess must be drained. Following the resolution of an appendix mass it is customary at a later date, i.e. 3–6 months later, to perform an appendicectomy. It is assumed that this will prevent further recurrence of appendicitis.

Gallbladder disease

Acute cholecystitis is a common cause of abdominal pain, particularly in the middle-aged patient. However, over the past few years it is becoming progressively more common in the younger female. This is probably associated with the contraceptive pill. Elective cholecystectomy is now the most frequently performed general surgical abdominal operation. Acute cholecystitis is caused by bacterial inflammation of the gallbladder wall, usually associated with gallstones. A typical attack of cholecystitis normally lasts 12–48 h. The character of the presentation of the attack will depend on whether there is obstructed drainage of the gallbladder. The majority of patients complain of progressive pain in the right hypochondrium associated with anorexia, nausea and vomiting. Where the gallbladder is initially obstructed, the pain may be very severe from the onset of the attack. Initially the patient may be managed at home with bed rest, pethidine 750–1000 mg 6-hourly, propantheline (Pro-Banthine) 30 mg qds and a broad-spectrum antibiotic. A cephalasporin is the drug of choice at the present time. On this regime the majority of patients will settle. However, those who fail to respond over a period of 24 h are best admitted to hospital. The subsequent management changes little, except that intravenous fluids are started, together with parenteral antibiotics.

Complications
An empyema or perforation of the gallbladder may develop and then immediate surgical intervention is required.

Subsequent management
A cholecystogram is performed to confirm the diagnosis, and usually 6 weeks later a cholecystectomy carried out. At this stage the inflammatory process will have resolved and in the majority of cases cholecystectomy may be performed without difficulty.

Immediate cholecystectomy
The indications for an immediate cholecystectomy are that the patient should be experiencing his or her first attack of cholecystitis and that there should be an experienced surgeon available to perform the operation. The oedema associated with the inflammation of the gallbladder makes removal of the gallbladder from the liver bed relatively easy. The patient also benefits in that, overall, his or her inpatient stay in hospital is reduced.

In patients who have had recurrent attacks of cholecystitis, the gallbladder is often fibrotic and small and cholecystectomy during the attack may be a very difficult operation. It is for this reason that immediate cholecystectomy is not advisable in this group of patients.

Diverticular disease

Diverticular disease is now one of the commonest conditions seen in a general surgical outpatient department. Diverticular disease in itself is relatively asymptomatic. It is the complications of the condition which gives rise to the acute abdomen. The severity of the symptom can depend upon the progression of the inflammatory process. Initially this starts as pericolic inflammation, and may go on to abscess formation and a generalized

42

peritonitis. Pyrexia, malaise and lower abdominal pain are the major symptoms. Examination reveals guarding and tenderness mainly in the left iliac fossa. The spread of the infection to the bladder may give rise to frequency of micturition or dysuria. Rectal examination may reveal a boggy mass in the pouch of Douglas. This is usually not a pelvic abscess but the inflamed oedematous sigmoid loop. In the early stages of the inflammation, the patient may be treated at home with broad spectrum antibiotics, such as Amoxil, Septrin, or a cephalasporin. The majority of patients will settle satisfactorily with this treatment. Patients who fail to settle may require more aggressive intravenous antibiotic therapy which usually includes a cephalosporin and metronidazole.

Indications for operation — Indications for operation are large bowel obstruction or evidence of an increasing peritonitis.

Operations — There are several operations used in the treatment of this condition. These are:

(1) A three-stage procedure involving initially a transverse colostomy followed by hemicolectomy and subsequent closure of transverse colostomy.

(2) A Hartmann's procedure which involves an initial resection of the abscess together with the inflamed descending and sigmoid colon. The proximal end of the colon is brought to the surface as an end colostomy and the distal end is closed and buried. At a later date – usually 2–4 months later – the colon is reanastamosed.

(3) A Paul–Mikulicz operation – this is particularly suitable where the sigmoid colon is involved. The sigmoid colon is mobilized and resected and the proximal and distal ends brought to the surface as a double-barrelled colostomy. This is then closed at a later date. This last operation is particularly suitable in the elderly patient in that it avoids a second major operation.

Pancreatitis

Acute pancreatitis — Diagnosis of acute pancreatitis is almost impossible to make without the confirmation of a raised serum amylase, i.e. greater than 1000 Somogyi units. The symptoms and signs may simulate those of acute cholecystitis or a perforated peptic ulcer. Alcoholism or previous epigastric pain are important pointers in the patient's history. It is not uncommon, as the condition

43

proceeds, for the patient to become mildly jaundiced. This is due to the oedema and inflammation in the head of the pancreas compressing the lower end of the common bile duct. Hospital treatment is required and, although in the early stages the patient may not look especially unwell, it is a condition with a mortality between 5 and 20%. Standard treatment involves intravenous fluid. The stomach is kept empty by nasogastric suction. A broad spectrum antibiotic is thought to be advisable. Glucagon appears to reduce the pain; the use of Trasylol at the present time is once again in doubt. A significant drop in the serum amylase level and low PO_2 are poor prognostic signs. At the present time there is no operative treatment suitable for acute pancreatitis. However, if there is doubt about the diagnosis and the possibility of an intra-abdominal perforation arises, a laparotomy should be performed. This does not appear to influence the prognosis in patients who turn out to have an underlying pancreatitis.

Later management

In order to avoid recurrent attacks, alcohol is to be avoided and a low fat diet advised. Since there is a high association between gallstones and pancreatitis, a cholecystogram should be performed. If a non-functioning gallbladder or gallstones are found a cholecystectomy should be performed.

Renal colic

In the case of renal colic, the classical clinical picture of a sudden onset of severe pain starting in the loin, spreading downwards to the groin and later radiating into the testis or labium usually presents little difficulty in diagnosis.

Obstructive causes

Large bowel obstruction

This usually presents little in the way of diagnostic difficulty. The two common causes of large bowel obstruction are carcinoma of the colon and diverticular disease. The less common causes include volvulus of the large bowel and pseudo large bowel obstruction.

Helpful diagnostic points

There is a number of diagnostic pointers.

Slow progressive abdominal distension in an otherwise well patient can be presumed to be due to an underlying colonic carcinoma. *Increasing left iliac fossa tenderness* associated with progressive distension is more likely to be due to a peri-

Abdominal distension

colic abscess secondary to diverticular disease. However, a

perforated carcinoma of the sigmoid colon may also present in a similar manner. *Asymmetrical abdominal distension* may be associated with an underlying volvulus of the colon.

Investigations Plain X-ray of the abdomen, sigmoidoscopy and rectal examination are the three most useful investigations in large bowel obstruction. An *abdominal X-ray* will confirm a suspected diagnosis of large bowel volvulus. It will also confirm the diagnosis of large large bowel distension and give useful information as to the possible level of obstruction. *Rectal examination* may reveal a palpable rectal carcinoma or even a frozen pelvis. In the elderly, it is surprising how often a patient with faecal impaction is initially diagnosed as having large bowel obstruction. *Sigmoidoscopy* – blood and mucus in the rectum will be strongly suggestive of an underlying carcinoma. Mucus and pus may be seen in a pericolic abscess.

The finding of a dilated rectum with the passage of excessive flatus may occur in *pseudo large bowel obstruction*. This is an important finding and may save the patient an unnecessary operation.

Treatment Treatment of large bowel obstruction resulting from diverticular disease and treatment of that resulting from carcinoma are very similar and has previously been discussed, under Diverticular disease.

A *colonic volvulus* involves either the caecum or the sigmoid colon. The only definitive treatment is to resect that portion of the colon involved in the volvulus. Unwinding the volvulus, deflating the bowel and tacking the colon back into place unfortunately only lead to a recurrence at a later date.

Small bowel obstruction

The common causes of small bowel obstruction in adults are (1) abdominal adhesions and (2) inguinal and femoral hernias.

The common presenting symptoms of small intestinal obstruction will include abdominal pain, vomiting, visible peristalsis, distension, dehydration and clinical shock. In the majority of patients the symptoms and signs develop progressively and often quite slowly. A subacute phase may be seen which may lead to complete small bowel obstruction but often may resolve spontaneously.

Diagnosis Usually there is little difficulty in making a diagnosis. The most useful investigation is a straight abdominal X-ray to reveal multiple small bowel fluid levels. *Sudden acute small bowel obstruction* occurs in small bowel obstruction associated

45

with gangrene of the small bowel. It is most commonly associated with abdominal adhesions in which the blood supply to the small bowel becomes rapidly occluded and gangrene develops. Severe, agonizing abdominal pain in a restless distressed patient may be mistaken for *renal colic* or *biliary colic*. The haemorrhagic exudate from *gangrenous small bowel* is extremely irritant and when the distress of a patient appears to be out of proportion to the abdominal findings, always suspect underlying gangrenous intestine as the cause.

Treatment   Where the small bowel is completely obstructed or the symptoms and signs suggest an underlying gangrenous small bowel, surgical intervention is mandatory. However, many patients who are subacutely obstructed will respond to intravenous fluid therapy and nasogastric aspiration. This small group will initially respond to conservative treatment but on subsequent oral feeding will once again develop the symptoms of subacute obstruction. The findings in this group of patients at laparotomy include partial obstruction due to adhesion, internal hernias and, occasionally, a Richter's hernia.

Perforations

Diagnosis   A generalized peritonitis with an X-ray finding of free air under the diaphragm is diagnostic of an intestinal perforation.

The following points may be helpful in making the diagnosis as to the site of the perforation: (1) a history of indigestion or previous peptic ulceration associated with severe epigastric pain strongly suggests a perforated gastric or duodenal ulcer; (2) a history of diverticular disease, constipation or a change in bowel habit associated initially with severe left iliac fossa pain suggests a perforation of the descending colon, common causes being diverticular disease, carcinoma or stercal ulceration.

The diagnosis of acute perforation of the small bowel is extremely difficult to make. The perforation is usually caused by a foreign body such as a meat or fish bone. However, these are rarely seen on X-ray.

Investigations   An abdominal X-ray in the erect position is the most useful investigation. The finding of free air under the diaphragm is diagnostic of an intestinal perforation. However, this sign will be absent in a small proportion of cases with an intestinal perforation. An important differential diagnosis is acute pancreatitis. *Perforation into the lesser sac of the stomach* is a difficult diagnosis to make and is often a surprise finding at

46

laparotomy. An X-ray of the abdomen in the erect and lateral positions may reveal gas behind the stomach.

Treatment

Perforated gastric ulcer

The commonly performed procedure is direct oversewing of the ulcer. The peritoneal soiling and local oedema usually make any definitive procedure impossible.

Perforated duodenal ulcer

Again the commonly performed procedure is direct suture of the ulcer. However, since the incidence of recurrence of a duodenal ulcer is high, a definitive procedure should be performed where possible. This is usually a bilateral truncal vagotomy and gastro-jejunostomy.

Perforation of small bowel

If the perforation is small it may be possible to directly oversew the perforation. However, a small bowel resection is usually necessary.

Perforation of colon

Treatment is similar to those procedures discussed for large bowel obstruction. Until a few years ago, faecal peritonitis was inevitably a fatal condition. Mortality has now been markedly reduced by the use of peritoneal lavage combined with an intravenous cephalosporin and metronidazole.

Gynaecological problems

Pelvic inflammatory disease (salpingitis)

A vaginal discharge associated with bilateral suprapubic tenderness and pain on cervical motion, represents the classic description of pelvic inflammatory disease. However, in many instances the vaginal discharge is absent. Right-sided salpingitis is often impossible to differentiate from acute appendicitis on abdominal examination.

Laparoscopy   Laparoscopy is useful in the diagnosis of salpingitis, but it is not used routinely. It has little place in the diagnosis of appendicitis, as the appendix cannot usually be visualized with the laparoscope. Where doubt exists between salpingitis and appendicitis, it is usually wiser to proceed to an appendicectomy and inspect the tubes and ovaries at the same time.

Ectopic pregnancy

In the average practice, ectopic pregnancies are considerably less common than appendicitis and pelvic inflammatory disease. Most mistakes arise because the diagnosis is not considered.

Classical presentation

The presenting signs and symptoms of an ectopic pregnancy will depend on the degree and rate of bleeding. Patients fall into one of two categories – those with the more classical signs and those in whom the diagnosis is not initially obvious.

A history of a missed period or an irregularity of periods, together with lower abdominal tenderness and a boggy mass in the pouch of Douglas, strongly suggests an ectopic pregnancy.

Subacute presentation

In subacute presentation there is an intermittent leak, the signs of which may be very similar to those of appendicitis. There is usually a history of a missed or an irregular period. Vaginal bleeding may or may not be present. Where there is any doubt between the diagnosis of appendicitis and that of an ectopic pregnancy, it is wise to assume the patient has an ectopic pregnancy until proved otherwise.

Intra-abdominal bleeding

Massive intra-abdominal bleeding is a life threatening condition which requires urgent treatment. When seen in the acute stage there is no doubt about the patient having an underlying peritonitis. This is caused by the massive irritation from the intra-abdominal blood. However, later the signs change and the abdomen becomes soft and doughy. It is at this stage that the diagnosis may be missed. The general appearance of the patient, together with a low blood pressure, thready pulse, and a distended abdomen should strongly suggest an underlying ectopic pregnancy.

Treatment

Where there is no doubt about the diagnosis, a laparotomy should be performed, and the necessary tubal surgery undertaken. Where there is doubt, a laparoscopy would confirm the diagnosis. If laparoscopy is not available, then an exploratory laparotomy is indicated.

Less common diagnoses

Aortic aneurysm

The majority of aortic aneurysms occur in the abdominal aorta below the renal arteries and above the aortic bifurcation. An

48

expanding aortic aneurysm is felt most easily in the left upper quadrant of the abdomen. Prior to rupture, the symptoms experienced by the patient are mainly attributable to the direct pressure effects of the aneurysm. These include backache, loin pain, which may simulate sciatica, renal colic and testicular disease, particularly on the left side. The symptoms and signs of a leaking aortic aneurysm will depend upon the site of rupture, i.e. intraperitoneal or extraperitoneal.

Intraperitoneal rupture

This catastrophic condition is characterized by sudden onset of severe central abdominal pain associated with a rapid drop in blood pressure followed quickly by death. Only a small proportion of ruptured aortic aneurysms bleed directly in to the abdominal cavity. The majority bleed initially extraperitoneally.

Extraperitoneal rupture

Pain is the most significant symptom in all patients with an extraperitoneal rupture of an aortic aneurysm. This is unrelenting and is often accompanied by a drop in blood pressure. What happens next in a patient will depend upon the size of the leak and the amount of blood lost. Those with a large retroperitoneal blood loss will remain hypotensive and eventually die. Rapid surgical intervention presents the patient with a small chance of survival. Where the initial blood loss is small, only a short period of hypotension may occur. Several hours or even days may intervene before further bleeding ensues. *Therefore any middle-aged or elderly male who collapses with abdominal pain should be assumed to have an aortic aneurysm until proved otherwise.*

Factors influencing survival

Factors influencing the survival of patients with ruptured aortic aneurysm include the general medical condition of the patient prior to the rupture, the experience of the operating surgeon and good postoperative intensive care facilities. However, the one factor which appears to be *most important* is the time which elapses between the initial rupture and the subsequent operative repair. Why should this be so?

In those patients who survive the operation but subsequently die in the postoperative period, there are two main causes of death: (1) respiratory failure and (2) renal failure.

49

The renal failure can be attributed to the extent of pre-operative hypotension. The respiratory failure is often associated with the shock–lung syndrome. The shock–lung syndrome is directly related to the volume of transfused blood given during the operation.

Operative mortality

This varies from 30 to 50%. The patients who fare best are those who are operated on quickly by an experienced local vascular surgeon. The transfer of patients from one hospital to another increases the overall mortality.

Operative treatment

Most ruptured aortic aneurysms can be repaired with a simple inlay Dacron tube graft. Where the common iliac arteries are also involved, a bilateral aorto-iliac or aorto-femoral graft becomes necessary.

Ischaemic bowel disease

The two blood vessels involved in ischaemic bowel disease are the superior and inferior mesenteric arteries. The cause of the ischaemia may be embolic or thrombotic secondary to atherosclerosis.

Inferior mesenteric artery occlusion

An occlusion of the inferior mesenteric artery will produce ischaemic necrosis of the descending and sigmoid colon. The extent of the necrosis will depend upon the secondary blood supply along the marginal artery of the colon from the supra-mesenteric artery.

The clinical pictures include pain and tenderness in the left iliac fossa followed 12–24 h later by bloody diarrhoea or blood-stained stool. In the majority of patients, symptoms resolve spontaneously. The diagnosis is often confused with diverticular disease. A subsequent barium enema may show the classical thumb print sign in the colon or, in severe cases, stricture formation. Only a small proportion of patients will require a colonic resection in the acute phase.

Superior mesenteric artery occlusion

The severity of the small and large bowel necrosis will depend on the site of the initial occlusion. If this occurs at the origin of the superior mesenteric artery, most of the small bowel and part of the large bowel will become necrotic. Segmental occlusion, however, will cause necrosis of a limited part of the intestine.

Clinical features
The majority of patients are elderly and may have atrial fibrillation. Signs of a generalized peritonitis in a distressed patient who is unable to lie still are characteristic of ischaemic necrosis of the intestine. The bloodstained fluid from necrotic intestine is exuded into the peritoneum and usually causes the patient great distress.

Operative treatment
If a localized segment of the intestine is involved, a resection and anastamosis may be possible. Complete involvement of the small bowel and part of the colon requires massive resection and anastamosis. In the majority of cases, the resulting short intestine is incompatible with life.

Medical causes

Although there are numerous medical causes for an acute abdomen, they are in practice extremely rare. The commonest medical condition mistaken for an acute abdomen is *lower lobe pneumonia*. The pain is usually exacerbated by respiration. The patient is often dyspnoeic. Diagnosis should be obvious from examination of the chest. However, in a number of patients it is not clear until a chest X-ray examination is performed.

Less commonly, *myocardial infarction* may give rise to epigastric pain and when accompanied by vomiting this may deepen confusion. A helpful clue in such patients is the absence of abdominal tenderness. The ECG will confirm the diagnosis in approximately 80% of cases.

Ketoacidosis due to uncontrolled or undiagnosed diabetes mellitus is commonly accompanied by profuse vomiting, severe abdominal pain and signs of peritonism. *Therefore all patients presenting with an 'acute abdomen' should have their urine examined for glucose and ketones.*

Recurrent abdominal pain and discomfort

Symptoms and diagnosis – Investigation

It is frequently necessary to investigate many patients who complain of recurrent abdominal pain or discomfort. However, attention to the history will often make the diagnosis obvious and lead to more logical and fruitful approach. It is particularly important to note the nature, severity, frequency and duration of each bout. It must be ascertained whether the pain is localized to a single site or diffuse and whether there is radiation to other areas. Finally, what are the particular factors that precipitate or relieve the symptoms?

Symptoms and diagnosis

Relationship to food | Many patients relate their abdominal pain or discomfort to eating and drinking. This is usually the predominant feature of so-called _dyspepsia_. The term is confusing, however, because it is also often used to describe other food-related symptoms, such as heartburn, dysphagia, regurgitation, abdominal distension, nausea and vomiting. The commonest causes of abdominal pain that have some relationship to eating and drinking are peptic ulcer, the irritable bowel syndrome and gastric cancer. Oesophagitis, due to gastro-oesophageal reflux, although mainly causing retrosternal pain, may give rise to pain high in the epigastrium (see Chapter 1, Heartburn). Considerably less common, but nevertheless well established, causes are mesenteric angina, Crohn's disease and pancreatic disease.

53

Although pain from all these conditions is often related to meals, the association is not invariable. Other conditions which give rise to abdominal pain and discomfort, but which are even more tenuously related to food intake, are gastritis, gallstones, aerophagy, psychological stress and depression.

Peptic ulcer

Peptic ulcer pain is usually experienced in the epigastrium. More rarely the maximum pain occurs in the hypochondria, usually the right. It is typically well localized, but may radiate retrosternally or to the back. Each attack characteristically lasts for a few minutes to 1 or 2 hours. It is relieved by food, milk, antacids or vomiting. In some patients food may precipitate pain but in a substantial proportion there is no relationship of symptoms to meals. The patient describes the symptoms as pain and not merely a discomfort. The descriptions most commonly used are 'knife-like' and 'gnawing'. *Waking in the early hours because of the pain is the feature which best distinguishes it from other conditions.* Bouts of pain commonly last for several weeks. This is then followed by complete remission of symptoms which may last for many months. Although some patients can relate onset of symptoms or relapse to stress and emotional disturbance, there is usually no clear association with these factors. *It is not possible to distinguish between duodenal and gastric ulcer on clinical evidence alone.*

Gastric carcinoma

Pain caused by stomach cancer also tends to be epigastric and cannot easily be distinguished from that of peptic ulcer. However, the characteristic periodicity and long history of peptic ulcer pain is absent. Unfortunately, antacids and other ulcer treatments often relieve the early symptoms. As the lesion advances pain becomes more persistent and this sequence of events should always raise suspicion, particularly in patients over the age of 40. Another common symptom is fullness in the upper abdomen which comes on after only a few mouthfuls of food. *Excessive weight loss due to profound anorexia* is certainly the most striking accompanying feature of gastric cancer. In contrast, weight loss in peptic ulcer when present is usually slight and results from a self-imposed diet or fear that food may induce pain. *Previous gastric surgery undoubtedly predisposes to gastric cancer.* Thus, the recurrence of dyspeptic symptoms and anorexia coming on many years after such an operation should alert the practitioner to this possible development. Examination may elicit only tenderness in the epigastrium as in peptic ulcer, but a mass may also be present. Enlarged cervical lymph nodes, ascites and pelvic secondaries palpable on rectal examination, indicate widespread inoperable disease.

54

The irritable bowel syndrome

The most helpful diagnostic feature of pain in the irritable bowel syndrome is the relationship to defaecation. There is frequently a feeling of generalized distension of the abdomen which, together with the pain, is eased by passing stool or flatus. In a smaller group, abdominal pain is briefly exacerbated by passing stool. Unfortunately, the relationship of pain to defaecation is not invariable in this condition. Characteristically, there is an associated history of alternating constipation and diarrhoea or frequency of defaecation (see p. 100).

The commonest site of pain in the irritable bowel syndrome is the lower abdomen. In some patients, however, the pain may be experienced predominantly in the hypochondria and epigastrium. The site may fluctuate during an attack and from one episode to another. In general the patient is less specific about the nature and site of pain than are patients with peptic ulcer. Terms such as 'bruised', 'burning', 'cramping' and 'colicky' are commonly used. Although some patients experience severe pain, many admit that the symptom is discomfort rather than pain. It rarely wakes them from sleep. Frequently symptoms are brought on by meals, and in these cases distinction from peptic ulcer is difficult. Similarly, pain arising from the hepatic flexure may be mistaken for recurrent cholecystitis. Frequently a diagnosis of recurrent appendicitis, and less often one of Crohn's disease, is made in those patients whose pain is predominantly in the right iliac fossa due to 'spasm' in the caecum. Pain in the left iliac fossa from 'spasm' of the sigmoid colon is often labelled as diverticulitis. It is difficult to make the correct diagnosis if the patient is seen during the first attack of his or her irritable bowel syndrome. However, cholecystitis, diverticulitis and appendicitis usually cause more severe pain and are accompanied by guarding, pyrexia and constitutional disturbance. The long history of erratic bowel habit and relationship of pain to defaecation are useful clues in more chronic cases.

Mesenteric angina

Ischaemia of the intestine is a rare cause of recurrent abdominal pain which, because it is exacerbated by meals, may be mistaken for peptic ulcer. It is most common in the elderly, and arterial disease is usually present elsewhere. Actual infarction may supervene, giving rise to diarrhoea and bleeding.

Pancreatic disease

Severe acute pancreatitis presents as an acute abdomen and shock. It is unlikely to be confused with the conditions under discussion in this chapter. However, less severe attacks of pancreatitis may be the cause of recurrent bouts of epigastric pain which have to be distinguished from the other disorders considered in this chapter.

Characteristic radiation is to the hypochondria and back. Severity varies from mild discomfort to intense pain. It is most frequently described as boring or a deep ache. Food and, particularly, alcohol may precipitate pain. The duration of an individual attack is longer than that due to peptic ulcer and there is no significant benefit from antacids. Leaning forward or lying prone often helps but potent analgesics are commonly needed for complete relief. Between episodes of pain there may be complete absence of symptoms, although a persistent epigastric ache is not uncommon. In those patients where recurrent attacks have led to permanent impairment of pancreatic function, additional clinical features may aid the diagnosis. These include malabsorption and diabetes mellitus. Examination during an attack will reveal epigastric tenderness. In some cases a pseudocyst may be palpable in the epigastrium and slight jaundice with bile in the urine is common. Pancreatic cancer also causes pain similar to pancreatitis. There may be remissions and exacerbations, presumably due to bouts of secondary pancreatitis. With invasion of neighbouring tissue, the pain becomes persistent. Weight loss and anorexia are typical additional features.

Crohn's disease
It is not unusual for patients with Crohn's disease to have suffered with recurrent abdominal pain for several years prior to definitive diagnosis. The pain may vary from vague discomfort after food to symptoms suggestive of peptic ulcer. The mechanism in such cases is not clear. Despite intensive investigation, including barium studies and endoscopies, these patients defy diagnosis until more definite symptoms or signs arise. These include attacks of central abdominal colic and distension due to small bowel obstruction and the formation of an inflammatory mass.

Large bowel cancer
The first symptom of colorectal carcinoma may be abdominal discomfort. In tends to be persistent and poorly localized and has only a vague relationship to meals. Additional features of anorexia, weight loss, a palpable mass, either abdominal or rectal, and anaemia are frequently present.

Gastritis
The diagnosis of gastritis was often made in the past to explain recurrent epigastric pain, when radiology failed to show peptic ulceration. However, endoscopy has shown that there is no consistent correlation between mucosal appearances, histology and symptoms. It therefore seems likely that many cases of so-called radiologically negative dyspepsias have been wrongly attributed to gastritis. Nevertheless, some patients when examined by endoscopy for dyspeptic symptoms are found

to have severe inflammation of the gastric mucosa and no other abnormality of the upper gastrointestinal tract. It seems reasonable to accept gastritis as the cause of symptoms in these patients. This degree of gastritis is particularly common after gastric surgery and in those taking anti-inflammatory drugs for arthritis. Alcohol abuse commonly leads to abdominal discomfort. However, gastritis is not always present and the mechanism in such cases remains obscure.

Aerophagy
Air may be sucked into the stomach whilst eating. Those who are rapid eaters are especially prone to this problem. Heartburn sufferers often develop a habit of swallowing saliva to relieve their pain and excessive amounts of air may be sucked coincidentally into the stomach. Anxiety may also induce 'swallowing' of air to relieve tension. A number of patients who suffer from aerophagy are psychiatrically disturbed. It seems that some of the abdominal discomfort caused by this phenomena is due to distension of the stomach, because belching frequently brings relief. Much of the air, however, passes into the bowel and it is probable that some pain is due to distension of the colon.

'Stress dyspepsia'
Patients with peptic ulcer and the irritable bowel syndrome often notice an exacerbation of symptoms when emotionally stressed. There is also, however, a large group of patients with stress-induced abdominal pain and discomfort who have neither of the former conditions. The pain tends to be poorly localized and seldom nocturnal. It is variably related to meals and relief with antacids is inconsistent. Other non-gastrointestinal symptoms are frequently present. Headaches, lethargy and depression are especially common. The mechanism of the pain is obscure. It is possible that bowel motility is disturbed in some of these patients. However, because they do not have diarrhoea, frequency of defaecation or constipation, they are not usually included in the category of irritable bowel syndrome. Treatment of coexistent depression or removal of identifiable stress factors often leads to complete resolution of symptoms.

Gallbladder disease
Disease of the gallbladder causes abdominal pain, but there is rarely a close or consistent relationship to food. *Biliary colic* occurs when a gallstone passes from the gallbladder into the cystic or common bile duct. It is of sudden onset and felt most intensely in the epigastrium. 'Colic' is a poor description, because severity increases without remission, the peak being reached within 1–3 hours. Examination during the pain may elicit tenderness in the upper abdomen. Jaundice is sometimes present, or the patient may subsequently notice passing bile-stained urine and pale stool. If the stone falls back into the gall-

57

bladder or passes down the common bile duct into the duodenum the severe pain subsides within a few hours, although continuing discomfort for several days is common. Antacids give no benefit and potent analgesics are usually necessary. Repeated attacks may occur but can be distinguished from peptic ulcer by the sudden onset, greater intensity and longer duration of each individual episode of pain; furthermore, there is no response to antacids and the pain does not recur every day for several weeks, as with peptic ulcer.

Acute cholecystitis occurs when a gallstone fails to pass or disimpact from the cystic duct. Acute inflammation of the gallbladder frequently causes a single episode of severe upper abdominal pain with guarding (see p. 41). Less severe attacks, when recurrent, pose a problem and have to be distinguished from other causes of episodic pain. Recurrent cholecystitis leads to pain in the right hypochondrium and tenderness to palpation. Radiation of pain to the back and scapular region is common. The degree of pyrexia and systemic disturbance varies in severity and duration but, together with the pain, may last for a week or more.

In the past, numerous vague symptoms, such as right hypochondrial discomfort, belching, flatulence, 'fat intolerance' and heartburn, have been *wrongly* attributed to gallstones. These are equally common in patients with or without gallbladder disease. It has been estimated that 20% of the population over 60 have stones in the gallbladder, but only 35% of those with stones ever develop problems such as biliary colic, cholecystitis, cholangitis and obstructive jaundice, that can be definitely attributed to the calculi.

Pain from the liver
The common causes of chronic or recurrent pain in the liver are congestive cardiac failure and carcinomatosis. The latter results in pain only when the peritoneum is directly involved or the liver hugely expanded.

Renal pain
Recurrent pain due to stones impacting in the ureter is almost invariably felt most intensely in the loin. Typical radiation is to the groin or penis. Frank or microscopic haematuria is common. A plain abdominal X-ray and intravenous pyelogram are usually diagnostic.

Musculoskeletal pain
Prolapsed intervertebral discs and other musculoskeletal disorders of the spine may cause recurrent abdominal pain by compressing thoracic and lumbar nerve roots. Symptoms in the back usually accompany the abdominal pain or discomfort and tend to be exacerbated and relieved by changes in posture. In a few patients hyperalgesia is present over the segment involved.

X-rays of the lumbar region often provide confirmatory evidence of a prolapsed disc or significant degenerative disease of the spine.

Investigation of recurrent abdominal pain and discomfort

It is clearly impractical to investigate every patient who presents at the surgery with abdominal pain or discomfort. However, by paying attention to the clinical features the practitioner will be able to adopt a logical approach and decide which patients need to be referred for investigation.

When peptic ulcer seems likely in the under-40 age group, it is reasonable to give an initial trial of antacid treatment. The patient should also be advised to stop smoking, stop drinking coffee and excessive amounts of alcohol and avoid any foods which precipitate his or her pain. Many will achieve good relief with this regime and use it again for subsequent attacks. It is probable that a significant proportion of the population have during a period in their lives, duodenal ulcers which are managed in this way and never confirmed by radiology or endoscopy. A large and seemingly increasing number will not be satisfied by this approach. This is often because symptoms are not adequately controlled and attacks become more frequent and severe. Alternatively, even though good symptomatic relief is achieved, they or their relatives press for objective confirmation of the diagnosis. Future management in such cases is probably helped by further investigation because it reassures the patient and also reinforces the doctor's line of management.

In patients over 40, in whom there is a greater risk that dyspeptic symptoms may be due to gastric cancer, investigation before treatment is usually advisable. This is particularly so in those who have had no previous abdominal symptoms and especially if there is accompanying anorexia, weight loss, anaemia or a raised erythrocyte sedimentation rate.

Barium meal is still the most widely used initial investigation. Providing the radiologist is experienced and a double contrast technique is employed, the great majority of significant lesions will be identified. Nevertheless, in practice, some duodenal ulcers and early gastric carcinomas are not detected. Thus, in 'X-ray negative' cases and if, for one of the reasons previously mentioned, a definitive diagnosis is considered necessary, upper gastrointestinal endoscopy should be arranged.

Endoscopy in some of these cases reveals upper gastrointestinal lesions but in others no cause for symptoms can be found. In this situation when organic disease is strongly suspected, it will be necessary to proceed to further investigation. When, however, the clinical picture suggests that stress or depression are important factors, reassurance, perhaps supported by appropriate drug therapy, should be given a trial at this stage. Inflammation of the duodenum (duodenitis) without ulceration is probably the commonest cause of abdominal pain missed on barium meal but confirmed by endoscopy. It seems likely it has the same symptomatology and aetiology as frank duodenal ulceration. The doubtful relevance of gastritis in abdominal pain has already been mentioned. Nevertheless, in post-gastrectomy subjects and those on anti-inflammatory agents complaining of epigastric pain, endoscopy may confirm gastritis as the cause of the problem. In the post-gastrectomy group it is not uncommon to see a recurrent ulcer at the anastomosis which the barium meal has not shown. Another group of patients commonly referred for endoscopy are those found to have a 'gastric ulcer' by the radiologist. Although the radiological features of cancer are frequently obvious, benign and carcinomatous ulcers may be confused. Endoscopic biopsy of the lesion, with follow-up after a course of treatment, is therefore advisable. Many gastroenterologists now proceed directly to endoscopy and dispense with the barium meal, but the former is not available on demand to most general practitioners.

Diagnosis of the irritable bowel syndrome is based upon the typical clinical features and by excluding other possible conditions. A suggested outline of investigation is discussed in Chapter 16.

A raised erythrocyte sedimentation rate and anaemia, in association with recurrent or chronic abdominal pain, suggests cancer or Crohn's disease. Despite sigmoidoscopy, rectal biopsy and barium studies, many cases of Crohn's disease will escape confirmation for several years. Diagnosis is often eventually made at laparotomy because the patient develops a mass or intestinal obstruction. More common use of the *colonoscope* in the future is likely to result in earlier diagnosis of Crohn's disease in many patients with unexplained abdominal pain. However, delay in diagnosing this condition does not appear to affect prognosis significantly. When colonic cancer is being considered, *positive faecal occult blood tests* should increase the suspicion. *Sigmoidoscopy and double contrast barium enema* are usually diagnostic. In a few cases when suspicion is high, but barium enema fails to support the diagnosis, colonoscopy will be necessary.

When abdominal pain is due to biliary colic or cholecystitis, an *oral cholecystogram* will usually demonstrate stones or a non-functioning gallbladder. The latter suggests there is a stone blocking the cystic duct. In many such patients, however, re-examination shows normal function of the gallbladder. Thus, before referral to the surgeon a repeat cholecystogram or an *intravenous cholangiogram* is indicated. Neither of these investigations is useful in the presence of jaundice because it prevents contrast media being excreted at sufficiently high concentrations. *Ultrasonic* examination is an alternative in this situation (see Chapter 11, Diagnosis of the common causes of jaundice). If seen during or soon after an attack, examination of the *urine may show bilirubin* and the *serum concentrations of bilirubin and alkaline phosphatase* are also frequently raised.

Patients suspected of having recurrent pancreatitis should have a *serum amylase* estimation during an attack of pain, even if this means attending the local emergency and accident department during unsocial hours. In patients who go on to develop chronic pancreatitis, 30% will have *calcification of the pancreas* visible on a plain abdominal X-ray. Other tests which are now commonly employed to confirm both inflammatory and neoplastic disease of the pancreas are *endoscopic retrograde pancreatography* (p. 89), *pancreatic function tests* (p. 89) and *ultrasound scanning.* Even when these investigations are used in combination, pancreatic disease is still often difficult to confirm. In this situation *laparotomy* is usually the next procedure. Unfortunately, pancreatic cancer, other than carcinoma of the ampulla of Vater, has an extremely poor prognosis. Thus, the main purpose in reaching an early definitive diagnosis is merely to avoid further unnecessary investigation.

5   Acute diarrhoea

Acute infective diarrhoea – Diarrhoea in travellers – Diarrhoea due to drugs

Acute infective diarrhoea

The most frequent cause of acute diarrhoea is infection of the alimentary tract and is covered by the term 'gastroenteritis'. In these cases the associated symptoms of nausea, vomiting, lassitude, headache, fever and shivering all point to infection as the cause of diarrhoea. Although there is usually no problem in making the diagnosis of infective gastroenteritis, the aetiological agent is only rarely identified. The illness is almost invariably shortlived. Therefore, *diarrhoea persisting without improvement for more than 2 weeks is unlikely to be due to infection.* In these patients the causes discussed in Chapter 6, Chronic and Recurrent Diarrhoea, should be considered.

Numerous species of bacteria are known to be pathogens, and more recently viruses have been implicated as an important cause of gastroenteritis, especially in children.

Toxin-induced diarrhoea

Staphylococcus aureus, Clostridia perfringens and some strains of *Escherichia coli* produce toxins which cause the small intestine to secrete large volumes of fluid. The colon is unable to compensate and watery diarrhoea results. Staphylococci and clostridia can cause diarrhoea without infecting the small intestine, because their toxins produced in contaminated food, prior to ingestion, are equally pathogenic. In contrast, *E. coli* have first to colonize the duodenum and jejunum before releasing toxins *in vivo*. Recent evidence suggests that the pathogenicity

63

of *E. coli* depends upon the capacity of certain strains to adhere to the small bowel epithelium. This prevents the removal of the organisms by peristalsis and allows toxin to accumulate in high concentration close to the epithelium. Symptoms coming on within 2–6 hours of eating contaminated food are likely to be due to preformed toxin. Vomiting is frequently the first of these and may be the dominant feature. It is followed within a few hours by profuse diarrhoea and central abdominal colicky pain. The disease is short lived and recovery is usually complete within 48 hours. Antibiotics are *not* indicated and, in view of the brief nature of the condition, antidiarrhoeal preparations are rarely required. The patient can usually maintain adequate hydration and nutrition with oral fluids. Very occasionally, toxin-induced diarrhoea may lead to sudden severe dehydration and circulatory collapse. This is particularly likely in the elderly, infants and those debilitated by other diseases. Such cases will need admission to hospital for intravenous therapy.

Salmonella   The commonest species of *Salmonella* causing enteritis in man is *S. typhimurium*, but many others have now been identified. It must be remembered that the disease caused by these organisms varies greatly from those due to *S. typhi* and *S. paratyphi*. Typhoid and paratyphoid are characterized by bloodstream and widespread tissue invasion. Diarrhoea is *not* usually the main feature.

The exact mechanism whereby salmonella cause diarrhoea is not understood. However, in contrast to staphylococcal and clostridial toxin-induced disease, physical disruption and invasion of the intestinal epithelium occur. The ileum is the most severely affected, but in some cases a colitis is also seen. Some strains of *E. coli* that do not produce enterotoxin may also cause diarrhoea by a similar mechanism. Infection usually results from contact with infected animals, meat, especially poultry, and dairy products. Food may also be contaminated by human carriers. The incubation period is between 12 and 24 hours, which helps to distinguish it from toxin-produced diseases. Symptoms include copious diarrhoea, often with blood and mucus, abdominal pain and vomiting. Accompanying fever and constitutional disturbance is common. Severe symptoms subside within 2–3 days but disturbed bowel habit may persist for 2–3 weeks. A fluid diet, antidiarrhoeal (codeine phosphate, loperamide, and kaolin and morphine) and spasmolytic drugs (mebererine and anticholinergics) help to keep the patient comfortable. Antibiotics are *rarely* indicated. The indiscriminate use of antibiotics in uncomplicated cases does nothing to shorten the course of the disease and may prolong the carrier state. Ampicillin or co-trimoxazole may, however, be needed for the rare case of severe infection which has led to prolonged constitutional disturbance and when bloodstream invasion has occurred.

Shigella dysentery

Shigella sonnei and *flexneri* are by far the commonest causes of bacillary dysentery in the British Isles. The more severe disease caused by the dysenteriae species is usually contracted overseas. Infection spreads by contact with infected stool or articles that a patient has handled or worn, rather than from contaminated food or water. Outbreaks in schools or other institutions are common. The incubation period is 2–4 d. The main symptom is diarrhoea accompanied by blood and mucus. Lower abdominal pain, tenesmus, anorexia, vomiting and headache are also common. Examination reveals a mild to moderate pyrexia and diffuse abdominal tenderness without guarding. Because the large intestine is predominantly affected, an inflamed rectal mucosa on proctoscopy can be helpful in reaching a diagnosis. The disease is usually self-limiting and a fluid diet and symptomatic treatment are all that are required. Antibiotics do not appear to reduce symptoms or eradicate the species of organism encountered in the British Isles and may propagate resistant strains. Admission to hospital is only necessary when dehydration threatens to lead to circulatory collapse and renal failure. Social conditions may also make domiciliary care impractical. However, when outbreaks occur in residential institutions it is probably wise to remove the initial victims. If the epidemic is uncurbed, further evacuation is not indicated.

Campylo-bacter

Only in the past 10 years has the genus *Campylobacter* been implicated as a cause of enteritis. It is a vibrio-like organism. The exact mechanism by which diarrhoea is induced remains unclear, but it seems likely these organisms have the capacity to invade the gut mucosa. The small intestine is the principal site involved but a colitis may occur. Many animals harbour *Campylobacter* – including chickens, sheep, pigs, dogs and cats. Unpasteurized milk and untreated water have been implicated in some outbreaks. It is now the most commonly identified cause of adult infective enterocolitis in the British Isles. Unlike most enteric infections there is an incubation period of several days and diarrhoea is frequently preceded for 24–48 h by prodromal symptoms. These are most commonly headache, myalgia, abdominal pain, pyrexia and shivering. Diarrhoea lasts for 2–3 d and is almost invariably accompanied

65

by severe colicky abdominal pain. The stool is watery and sometimes contains blood. Lassitude and recurrent colic may persist
for several weeks.

In a small number of cases the severity of abdominal pain
and tenderness leads to an incorrect diagnosis of peritonitis and
laparotomy. In others, systemic disturbance, including arthritis,
predominates. Fortunately, most patients require only symptomatic management. The place of antibiotics is not clear, but they
should probably be reserved for the more severe cases. Erythromycin is the first choice.

Apart from shigellosis, bacterial diarrhoea is not usually
transmitted from person to person. Because the pathogen is
frequently contained in food, many individuals may be affected
simultaneously. When such outbreaks occur it is often possible
to trace the origin of the contaminated food.

Virus   Virus infections of the gut tend to occur in epidemics.
infections Schools and other similar institutions are particularly
vulnerable, presumably because transmission of the organism is
facilitated under these conditions. Many viruses have been
implicated in epidemics of gastroenteritis but the two most
consistently involved are rota-viruses and parvovirus-like
organisms, which include the Norwalk agent. The former are
almost certainly the commonest cause of childhood gastroenteritis in temperate climates.

As with the great majority of acute bacterial diarrhoeas,
viral enteritis in adults is a shortlived disease and requires no
more than domiciliary symptomatic management in most cases.

Diarrhoea in travellers

Travellers' All of the above bacterial causes of diarrhoea may be con-
diarrhoea   tracted in the British Isles but are more common in those
countries where standards of hygiene and sanitation are poor.

It seems very likely that pathogenic *E. coli* are the
commonest cause of diarrhoea in travellers to foreign countries,
whether it be to Spain, Central America or the Middle East. The
disease usually occurs within the first 2 weeks of arriving in the
new country. Because it lasts for only 2–3 days most individuals
have recovered by the time they return home. Prophylactic
Streptotriad, one tablet twice daily, reduces the incidence of
this disease. If the disease is more prolonged and persists after
returning then shigella, salmonella or parasitic infestation
should be considered.

66

Acute diarrhoea

Giardia
lamblia

By far the most likely parasite to cause acute diarrhoea in travellers is *Giardia lamblia*. It is endemic in the tropics, subtropical regions and the eastern Mediterranean. Outbreaks have also occurred in the USA and visitors to the USSR, particularly Leningrad, often return with this infestation. The organism is a flagellate protozoon which lives in human small intestine. Cysts are excreted in stool and infection occurs by ingesting contaminated food or water. Infestation is often asymptomatic; in those with symptoms there is a wide range of severity. Intermittent diarrhoea with abdominal discomfort and distension is common. In more severely affected cases the diarrhoea is profuse and significant malabsorption with weight loss can occur. Diagnosis is confirmed by the findings of cysts in the stool. Because these are not always present, examination of the duodenal fluid for trophozoites may be necessary to prove the diagnosis. Aspiration of duodenal fluid is usually combined with small bowel biopsy, sections from which will often reveal the organism between the villi. In severe cases there may be a mucosal abnormality with partial villous atrophy similar to that of tropical sprue.

Treatment is with metronidazole (Flagyl) 200 mg tds for 2 weeks, or 400 mg tds for 1 week. The patients should be warned not to take alcohol with metronidazol because the drug has Antabuse-like effect.

Amoebiasis

Infestation with *Entamoeba histolytica* is a rarer cause of diarrhoea in temperate climates than *Giardia lamblia*. Nevertheless, it is not exclusive to the tropics and is found in warm countries when sanitation and hygiene are poor. Infection occurs by ingestion of cysts which can contaminate water and food. The incubation period varies from a few weeks to several months. The disease may not manifest, therefore, until well after the patient has returned from his travels. In the majority of cases there is insidious onset of diarrhoea, the stool being mixed with blood and mucus. There is frequently no fever and only at a later stage does the patient complain of any systemic disturbance. Sigmoidoscopy shows scattered ulceration. Stool examination will reveal cysts and in fresh faeces it may be possible to see the motile trophozoites. Sections of a rectal biopsy should also be examined for trophozoites and the serum examined for antibodies to *E. histolytica*.

A small minority of patients have a more acute and severe disease. Their symptoms consist of bloody diarrhoea, fever and abdominal pain. Toxic dilatation of the colon is a rare complication in this group. Sigmoidoscopic appearances cannot be

67

distinguished from idiopathic ulcerative proctocolitis. A history of travel and the relevant investigations are, therefore, vital in making a rapid diagnosis in such cases.

If untreated, there may be spread of disease to cause an amoeboma or hepatic abscess. The most frequently used drugs are metronidazole and diloxanide furoate, which is particularly potent against cysts.

Other parasites Other parasitic infestations causing diarrhoea in patients returning to the British Isles are much less common. They include *Schistosoma mansoni*, tapeworms, *Ascaris lumbricoides*, hookworm, whipworm, *Trichinella spiralis* and *Strongyloides stercoralis*. In most cases examination of the stool will reveal the organism or its cysts. Sigmoidoscopy and rectal biopsy is particularly valuable in the diagnosis of schistosomiasis. When requesting stool examination for parasites, it is important to state the countries in which the patient has stayed – even though the visit may have been many years in the past – because these parasites have characteristic geographical distributions.

Tropical sprue must also be considered in those patients with diarrhoea returning from endemic areas. This condition is discussed in Chapter 7, Malabsorption.

Suggested guidelines in the management of infectious diarrhoea are as follows.

(1) Take stool, vomitus and suspected food to local microbiology laboratory.

(2) Advise fluid diet and prescribe antidiarrhoeal and spasmolytic drugs when necessary.

(3) Do not give antibiotics routinely.

(4) Emphasize importance of strict hygiene to patient and relatives.

(5) Admit to hospital if there is severe systemic disturbance, evidence of dehydration or other complicating disease.

(6) In infants, seek paediatrician's advice in all but the mildest cases.

(7) In cases where the organism has been identified, or where a common source of infection seems likely, notify the local health authority.

(8) Instruct anyone who handles food that they may not do so until their stools are free of the pathogen.

Diarrhoea due to drugs

Acute diarrhoea may be caused by drugs of many different categories. It is, therefore, very important to review current and recent drug regimes in any patient presenting with diar-

Antibiotic induced diarrhoea

rhoea. Other than laxatives, antibiotics are the therapeutic agents that most often cause this problem. Broad spectrum antibiotics are usually involved. Most patients have only mild bowel disturbance and the disorder usually passes within 2–3 days of stopping the antibiotic.

Pseudo-membranous colitis

The most serious form of antibiotic-induced diarrhoea is *pseudomembranous colitis*. This disorder, as its name implies, is an inflammatory disease of the large intestine. Sigmoidoscopy reveals the characteristic pseudomembrane overlying an oedematous hyperaemic mucosa. Histology shows areas of intense but superficial ulceration. The pseudomembrane consists of epithelial debris, fibrin and leukocytes. In the most severe cases, microthrombi and crypt abscesses are seen. The lesion is often patchy; a single biopsy, therefore, may not be representative. The diarrhoea consists of profuse liquid stool which sometimes contains blood. Other features, which include colic, pyrexia and leukocytosis, vary greatly in severity. In some cases intensive intravenous therapy is needed to correct dehydration, electrolyte imbalance and hypoproteinaemia. On rare occasions a toxic megacolon develops, which may necessitate colectomy. The symptoms can commence within the first few days of antibiotic treatment, but onset is more usual between the fourth and tenth days. It is, nevertheless, important to realize that symptoms may not start until 3 weeks after antimicrobial drugs have ceased. This latter group frequently have a more severe and protracted illness.

Many patients who develop pseudomembranous colitis have other debilitating diseases or have recently undergone surgery. It seems likely that a serious illness itself can be responsible for pseudomembranous colitis, because there have been a few documented cases in which antibiotics have not been involved.

The antibiotics most often implicated are clindomycin, lincomycin and ampicillin, but there have been sporadic reports which throw suspicion on many others.

The cause of this disease, in the great majority of cases, is a toxin produced by *Clostridium difficile*. It seems probable that antibiotic therapy either renders the colonic mucosa more vulnerable to the toxin or enhances the proliferation of *C. difficile* by reducing the numbers of other organisms. In many patients whose diarrhoea starts whilst on antibiotics, stopping the drug results in cure. In those whose symptoms start or persist after stopping the offending antibiotic, vancomycin, 150 mg four times daily, should be given.

In the past, *Staphylococcus aureus* was considered to be the cause of pseudomembranous enterocolitis. Proven staphylococcal enterocolitis is now very rare and it seems likely that many cases previously attributed to this organism were really due to *Clostridium difficile*. It is not known if the very common, mild and rapidly resolving attacks of antibiotic induced diarrhoea are also due to *C. difficile* toxin or whether other mechanisms are involved.

Other drugs causing diarrhoea
There can be few drugs that have not been blamed for causing diarrhoea. In the situation where symptoms have coincided with starting a new drug, it is wise where possible to stop it and change to an alternative preparation. Drugs that often cause diarrhoea include carbenoxylone and other liquorice derivatives, antacids containing magnesium salts, digoxin (at toxic levels) mephanamic acid (Ponstan), indomethazine (Indocid), guanethidine (Ismelin), colchicine and the majority of cytotoxic agents. In addition to causing diarrhoea some drugs may also cause malabsorption. Amongst these are neomycin, cholestyramine, phenindione and para-aminosalicylic acid.

Chronic and recurrent diarrhoea

Causes and indications – Investigations

There is no strict definition of diarrhoea, but the term is probably best restricted to describe excessive amounts of poorly formed stool. The definition of 'chronic' in such cases is not exact but includes those where the history is measured in weeks rather than days. In many cases there have been recurrent episodes over several years. This category, therefore, excludes most of the infective causes of bowel disease which have been dealt with in Chapter 5, Acute diarrhoea.

The patient's definition of diarrhoea may not coincide with that given above. Attention to what he or she is really describing is, therefore, of considerable importance. By combining this information with other clinical features and the results of relatively simple investigation, it will be possible to diagnose the cause of diarrhoea quickly in the majority of patients.

Causes and indications

The common causes of chronic or recurrent diarrhoea are the irritable bowel syndrome, inflammatory bowel disease (ulcerative colitis and Crohn's disease), carcinoma of the large intestine, malabsorption and gastric surgery. The first three conditions account for well over 90% of all cases of chronic or recurrent diarrhoea. The major part of the following discussion, therefore, compares and contrasts the clinical and investigative findings in these disorders.

71

Timing, amount and description

The passing of several unformed stools within the first hour after rising from bed is a characteristic feature of the irritable bowel syndrome. Many patients with this condition are only affected during this period and remain free of symptoms for the rest of the day. All forms of the irritable bowel syndrome may be exacerbated by stress and tension, but the group with morning diarrhoea seem to be particularly affected by these factors. Absence of symptoms at weekends is common. In others, there is an urgent call to pass stool within a few minutes of eating a meal. However, in many cases of the irritable bowel syndrome there is no fixed pattern. Diarrhoea due to inflammatory bowel disease (ulcerative colitis and Crohn's disease) may also be restricted to the morning, but usually has a less rigid temporal pattern. The need to pass stool during the night is very uncommon in the irritable bowel syndrome and usually indicates inflammatory disease.

Regular passage of large amounts of faeces, which is often of liquid consistency (greater than 400–500 ml per day), is indicative of widespread inflammatory disease of the colon or malabsorption. Some patients, especially those with the irritable bowel syndrome, although complaining of 'diarrhoea', are really suffering from frequency of defaecation. Characteristically, they pass small pellets or thin thread-shaped stools often weighing only a few grams. These patients also complain that the rectum feels full even after passing stool. This latter sensation is not, however, pathognomonic of the irritable bowel syndrome, as inflammatory disease of the rectum, rectal neoplasms and faecal impaction give rise to the same symptom.

Blood and mucus *mixed* with the stool are an indication of organic disease and are most likely to result from inflammatory disease of the large intestine, diverticular disease or neoplasia. Blood alone, particularly if present only on the toilet paper, is frequently caused by piles or an anal fissure, but this must *not* be assumed without adequate examination and appropriate investigation. Mucus but *not* blood may coat the stool in the irritable bowel syndrome. Mucus in large amounts, often passed in the absence of stool, may be caused by tumours or inflammation of the large intestine.

Steatorrhoea is usually described by the patient as diarrhoea. Further questioning will elicit that he or she is passing the characteristic pale, bulky and offensive stool that results from malabsorption of fat. Because of the high fat content it floats and is difficult to flush away. It should, nevertheless, be remembered that stool containing an excess of gas will also float and that floating stools do not, therefore, always indicate steatorrhoea.

'Silver' stools result from changed blood mixing with steatorrhoea. It is usually due to carcinoma of the pancreatic head.

Although a patient's description of the stool may be helpful, it is no substitute for examination of the faeces. This is obviously difficult but not impossible in general practice or the outpatient clinic. Nevertheless, because of the difficulty of obtaining an accurate assessment of bowel action and nature of the stool, it is often necessary to admit the patient to hospital for this purpose.

Alternating diarrhoea and constipation

A prolonged history of erratic bowel habit with episodes of diarrhoea, followed by periods of difficulty in moving the bowels, is characteristic of the irritable bowel syndrome. However, a similar history involving only weeks or a few months may indicate carcinoma of the large intestine.

Spurious diarrhoea

Many elderly and bedridden patients complain of passing liquid stool often with faecal incontinence. This is due to impaction of stool in the rectum with leakage of liquid around the solid faecal mass. The impaction is usually the result of generalized and rectal inertia. The problem is made worse by the taking of laxatives and can only be solved by clearing the rectum. This can sometimes be achieved with stool softeners (dioctyl sodium sulphosuccinate) and washouts. In many cases, only manual removal is successful. *Carcinoma of the rectum or left side of the colon may also cause spurious diarrhoea.*

Accompanying symptoms

Although diarrhoea may be the predominant symptom, additional attention should be paid to other clinical features, both in the history and on examination. By so doing, it may be possible to avoid unnecessary, expensive and time-consuming investigation.

Weight loss

Diarrhoea accompanied by weight loss, without severe anorexia, should raise the suspicion of malabsorption, due to either small bowel disease or pancreatic insufficiency. These two symptoms are also common in thyrotoxicosis. One or more of the other common features of thyrotoxicosis is usually present in such cases. These include irritability, insomnia, heat intolerance, palpitations, cardiac failure, amenorrhoea, tremor, exophthalmos, lid lag and a thyroid bruit.

Anorexia

When weight loss and diarrhoea are accompanied by anorexia, a search must be made for *carcinoma* of the large intestine. This triad of symptoms may also be found in Crohn's disease and depression. *They are always an indication for investigation.*

73

Abdominal
pain

The diarrhoea of the irritable bowel syndrome is painless in approximately 10% of patients. In a larger group, the bowel disturbance is accompanied by pain. This is most common in the lower abdomen but may also be experienced in the hypochondria and epigastrium. Some patients describe the pain as colic or cramp. In others there is a vaguer discomfort with the sensation of distension and bloating. Unfortunately, patients with Crohn's disease and carcinoma of the bowel may experience similar symptoms.

Travel

A history of travel overseas is important, particularly if recent. Infestation with *Entamoeba histolytica* and *Giardia lamblia* and tropical sprue particularly must be kept in mind.

Drugs and
alcohol

Enquiry should be made about proprietary medicines including laxatives and herbal preparations based on senna or liquorice and antidyspepsia mixtures containing magnesium salts. Unfortunately, some patients who take laxative preparations will not admit to doing so. Many of them have anorexia nervosa or some other psychological disturbance. Such patients are often subjected to extensive investigation before the true diagnosis is made (p. 93). Abuse of alcohol disturbs bowel function, but patients often refuse to attribute the diarrhoea to their drinking habits.

Physical
examination

Thorough examination of patients with persistent or recurrent diarrhoea is essential. Positive findings may indicate the need for laboratory or radiological tests and point to those investigations that are likely to be most fruitful. A routine examination that reveals no abnormality does not, of course, eliminate organic disease and if the history has already raised definite suspicions it will still be necessary to investigate.

A mass

Carcinoma of the large intestine, particularly of the right colon, and Crohn's disease of the terminal ileum and caecum often give rise to a palpable mass.

Tenderness
and guarding

Tenderness and definite guarding in the right iliac fossa in a patient with chronic recurrent diarrhoea suggests Crohn's disease. Diverticulosis of the large intestine often seems to accompany the irritable bowel syndrome, but whether this is greater than would be expected by chance is not clear. Diverticulosis will, nevertheless, in some cases develop into diverticulitis and if there is coexistent diarrhoea, due to the irritable bowel syndrome, it may be confused with Crohn's disease. Diverticulitis may give rise to tenderness and guarding anywhere in the lower abdomen. Tenderness on palpation may also occur in the irritable bowel syndrome *per se*. In these cases it is frequently possible to palpate a rigid pipe-like colon in the left iliac fossa which is due either to stool or spasm of the colonic muscle. Definite guarding, accompanied by pyrexia, indicates inflammation and favours the diagnosis of Crohn's disease or diverticulitis.

Rectal examination   Digital examination of the rectum is obligatory. Blood on the glove confirms the need for more extensive investigation, because of the possibility of either neoplastic or inflammatory bowel disease (p. 161). In many cases the site of bleeding will be piles or diverticular disease. Either of these conditions, when accompanying the irritable bowel syndrome can, therefore, be confused with more sinister pathologies such as carcinoma and inflammatory bowel disease (p. 161). The majority of rectal carcinomas can be felt within the lumen and many cancers of the sigmoid will also be palpable extrinsic to the rectal wall. Perianal fissures, fistulae and fleshy skin tags favour the diagnosis of Crohn's disease.

Anaemia   Clinical evidence of anaemia is against the diagnosis of the irritable bowel syndrome. Instead, one should be alerted to the distinct possibility of carcinoma, inflammatory bowel disease or small bowel malabsorption. The anaemia of small bowel malabsorption may be accompanied by other signs of malnutrition such as glossitis and angular stomatitis.

Oedema due to increased protein catabolism and *bone and muscle* pain, resulting from malabsorption of vitamin D, are rarer associated features of malabsorption.

Lymphadenopathy   A search for enlarged nodes is important. Large bowel carcinoma may metastasize to nodes in the supraclavicular fossae. Enlarged nodes elsewhere may be due to lymphoma which, when it involves the small intestine, commonly causes diarrhoea and steatorrhoea. Biopsy of the involved peripheral nodes in these situations will provide a rapid diagnosis and obviate unnecessary investigation.

Points to stress

- Frequency of defaecation restricted to the period soon after rising is usually due to the irritable bowel syndrome.

- Diarrhoea with weight loss, blood *per rectum* or anaemia requires early investigation.

- Rectal examination will diagnose a high proportion of colorectal cancers and lead to early surgical referral.

Investigation

Sigmoidoscopy Sigmoidoscopy must be performed in chronic diarrhoea. Endoscopy of the rectum can be carried out easily in the surgery or
outpatient clinic without need of bowel preparation. Only very
young children, the rare extremely anxious patient and those
with painful anal fissures require sedation or anaesthesia.
Sigmoidoscopy and biopsy will confirm the diagnosis of rectal
carcinoma. Examination of the mucosa *combined with biopsy*
will provide a definite diagnosis in virtually all cases of ulcerative proctocolitis and in many patients with Crohn's disease. In
ulcerative colitis, the rectum is uniformly involved. The lesion
ranges from hyperaemia and oedema to granularity in the mild
and moderately affected cases. In severe disease there is
spontaneous bleeding and disruption of the mucosa. When the
condition is restricted to the rectum, it may be possible to get
above the involved segment and view normal mucosa. Crohn's
disease frequently spares the rectum. In other cases of Crohn's
disease there are patches of inflammation and discrete ulceration. Aphthous-type ulcers of the rectal mucosa are also found in
this condition. A cobblestone appearance of the mucosa is
another characteristic feature of Crohn's disease. Amoebic
colitis cannot be distinguished readily from these two conditions
on naked eye appearances. Thus, those who have been to areas
where this disease is endemic must also have the appropriate
stool and serological tests. Even when no definite lesion can be
seen, blood or excessive mucus coming from above the endoscope indicates that there is need for continuing investigation.

Stool With the exception of *Mycobacterium tuberculosis* and
examination possibly *Shigella*, bacteria do not cause chronic diarrhoea.
Culture of fresh stool is advisable to exclude these pathogens
and is particularly necessary in immigrants. By contrast, infestation with *Entamoeba histolytica* commonly goes on to cause
chronic bowel disturbance. The former should be suspected in
patients from developing countries who complain of blood-
stained diarrhoeal stool. It is essential that fresh faeces are
examined when looking for pathogenic amoeba. A serological
test is now also available and is positive in a high percentage of
cases.

Another protozoon, *Giardia lamblia*, may also cause chronic
diarrhoea and sometimes steatorrhoea. It infests the small
intestine and it is, therefore, best confirmed by examination of
duodenal juice obtained by intubation. This procedure is often
combined with small bowel biopsy. Stool examination for the
Giardia lamblia ova is also positive in a smaller proportion of

patients. When making a request for stool examination and culture, it is important to include amongst the clinical data the countries to which the patient has been and whether there has been recent antibiotic treatment. A minimum of three stool samples should be supplied.

Occult bleeding

In patients with diarrhoea who give a history of blood loss and when none is found on rectal examination, a search should be made for occult blood in three separate stools. The 'Haem-occult' test is a newly available means of performing this investigation. It is particularly designed to detect large intestinal bleeding. The test is cheap and can be performed conveniently in the surgery or clinic without special apparatus. A positive result is likely to indicate inflammation of the bowel, diverticular disease or neoplasia, provided that an obvious cause such as piles or fissure has been excluded by proctoscopy.

Initial blood tests

A normal haemoglobin concentration and white cell count, together with an erythrocyte sedimentation rate in single figures, though not excluding organic disease, favours the diagnosis of the irritable bowel syndrome. A low haemoglobin in patients with diarrhoea may be the result of intestinal neoplasia, ulcerative colitis, Crohn's disease or small bowel malabsorption. The anaemia in neoplastic and inflammatory disease of the bowel is partly due to bleeding. If prolonged, this will result in an iron deficiency picture, with a low mean corpuscular volume and mean corpuscular haemoglobin concentration. Both conditions, however, may also be associated with the normo-chromic–normocytic anaemia of 'chronic disease'. Small bowel malabsorption is often accompanied by iron deficiency. A dimorphic blood film is also found in this condition due to combined deficiency of iron and folate or vitamin B_{12}.

In patients with chronic diarrhoea, a low serum albumin level is most likely to be due to excessive gut loss of protein. Active widespread inflammatory bowel disease is the commonest cause. It may also result from coeliac disease and small bowel lymphoma. In rare instances large amounts of protein can be lost from a large bowel carcinoma. Normal plasma protein levels are found in the irritable bowel syndrome.

When small bowel malabsorption is suspected because of the clinical features outlined above, the finding of low blood levels of folate and vitamin B_{12} would strengthen the suspicion and encourage definitive investigation (p. 81).

Further investigations

Prior to proceeding to radiological examinations, the possibility of endocrine disease as the cause of diarrhoea should be considered.

Thyrotoxicosis   Thyrotoxicosis causes diarrhoea by increasing small bowel motility and reducing the gut transit time. It is easily confirmed by estimation of serum tri-iodothyronine and thyroxine concentrations.

Diabetes mellitus   Diabetes mellitus is occasionally complicated by diarrhoea which is often nocturnal. The mechanism is not entirely clear but is probably partly due to an autonomic neuropathy of the gut leading to abnormal motility. There may be an alteration in gut bacterial flora and disturbance of bile salt metabolism. Treatment is frequently ineffective. Some patients respond to simple antidiarrhoeal agents and others benefit from courses of broad spectrum antibiotics. Recently cholestyramine, a substance which binds bile salts and interferes with their cathartic action on the intestine, has proved useful.

Carcinoid syndrome   The carcinoid syndrome is a very rare cause of diarrhoea. Carcinoid tumours of the small intestine, when they metastasize to the liver, can produce large quantities of 5-hydroxytryptamine, kallikrein and prostaglandins. These substances affect gut function and lead to diarrhoea which may be continuous or episodic. The accompanying features of flushing, dilatation of skin blood vessels, asthma and signs of pulmonary and tricuspid valvular disease of the heart support the diagnosis. Elevated levels of 5-hydroxyindolacetic acid in the urine are confirmatory. Treatment includes symptomatic relief with 5-hydroxytryptamine antagonists. In some cases it is possible to enucleate the secondary tumours from the liver. Cytotoxic drugs infused into the hepatic artery may also give symptomatic relief. The tumour is slow growing and 50% of patients can be expected to live for 5 years or longer from the time of presentation.

Radiology   Patients with chronic diarrhoea who also pass blood *per rectum* should be referred for a double contrast barium enema. Although many of these patients will have nothing more sinister than the irritable bowel syndrome, in association with piles, or diverticular disease, carcinoma and inflammatory bowel disease must be excluded. Even if these conditions have been confirmed by endoscopy, barium enema is still necessary. This is because in carcinoma of the rectum there may be other tumours beyond the range of the sigmoidoscope and in ulcerative colitis or Crohn's disease it is important to define the distribution of the inflammation.

In those cases where there is no evidence of bleeding and endoscopy has shown a normal rectal mucosa, but haematological tests have revealed anaemia or a raised erythrocyte sedimentation rate, radiology is also indicated. The likely diagnoses under these circumstances are colonic cancer or Crohn's disease. When the barium enema is normal, but Crohn's disease is still suspected, a barium follow-through examination of the small intestine should be arranged.

If there is no evidence of intestinal bleeding and the rectal biopsy, stool and blood tests are normal, the decision whether to arrange barium studies is more difficult. In patients over the age of 30 in this group, it is wise to proceed to a barium enema in order to exclude carcinoma. In those under 30 the barium enema is not so immediately vital, because cancer of the large intestine is extremely unlikely in this age group. It must be admitted that this plan of investigation will undoubtedly delay the diagnosis in a small number of patients with Crohn's disease. Nevertheless, it is extremely unlikely that these cases will be in jeopardy providing they are kept under review and investigated further if symptoms worsen or new signs develop. It is, therefore, important to keep an open mind about the final diagnosis in this group.

Colonoscopy   Colonoscopy is indicated in patients when investigation points to either large bowel carcinoma or inflammatory disease, but double contrast barium enema and sigmoidoscopy have failed to confirm the diagnosis. This procedure has now become widely available. The new fibre optic instruments make possible a thorough examination of the entire large bowel, and tissue can be obtained for histology. The colon must be clear of faeces; this can be achieved by a number of different techniques. Most centres combine a low roughage diet, purgation and colonic lavage. Parenteral sedation and analgesia are given immediately prior to the examination. As with upper gastrointestinal endoscopy, the patient is able to return home later the same day.

7 Malabsorption

Mechanisms of malabsorption – Clinical features – Investigation of suspected malabsorption

Malabsorption may result from a number of different mechanisms.

Mechanisms of malabsorption

1. Diffuse disease of small intestine

Diffuse disease of the small intestine, such as coeliac disease and tropical sprue, results in reduction of digestive and absorptive function of the epithelial cells.

2. Resection of small intestine

Resection of the small intestine because of trauma, inflammation, neoplasia or vascular disease, will reduce the total surface available for absorption. In health the great majority of carbohydrate, protein fat, vitamins and minerals are absorbed in the duodenum and jejunum. However, long sections of upper small bowel may be removed without causing significant malabsorption. This is because the small intestine has a large reserve capacity and the ileum is capable of actually increasing its absorptive function in response to jejunal resection or disease.

Vitamin B_{12} and bile salts are normally actively absorbed in the terminal ileum. Thus, removal or disease of this section of the small intestine, because of conditions such as Crohn's disease, will lead to specific problems. The most common is vitamin B_{12} deficiency which causes a macrocytic, megaloblastic anaemia. Bile salt malabsorption is another serious consequence. These substances are produced in the liver and pass via the biliary system into the duodenum. They act as detergents and allow the products of fat digestion to mix with water in the gut lumen. This involves the formation of aggregates called 'mixed micelles'. This process facilitates the absorption of fatty acids, monoglycerides and fat soluble vitamins from the duodenum and jejunum. The bile salts themselves are not absorbed at these sites but are released from the micelles into the lumen. This enables them to be reutilized, if necessary, throughout the length of the small intestine. They are eventually actively absorbed from the terminal ileum and pass via the circulation to the liver, from where secretion into the biliary system again takes place. This conservation is essential because the liver has a very limited capacity to synthesize bile salts. When bile salt absorption is impaired, due to disease or resection of the ileum, recirculation is interrupted. This causes bile salt deficiency with a reduction in micelle formation and malabsorption of fat and fat soluble vitamins. In this situation bile salts pass into the colon where they have a potent cathartic action. Such patients, therefore, suffer from both steatorrhoea and diarrhoea.

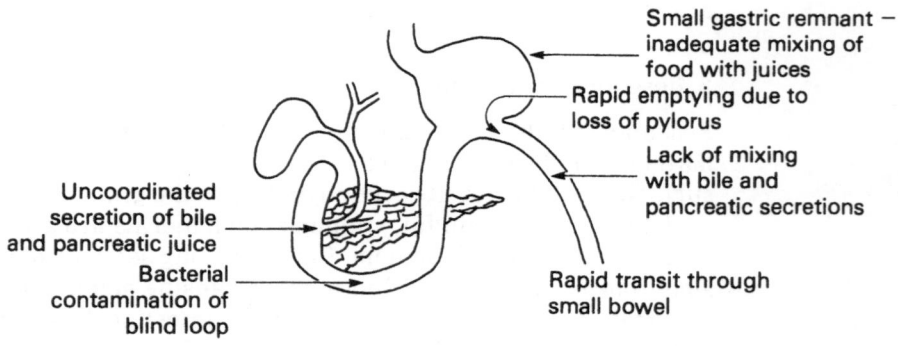

Causes of malabsorption after gastric surgery

Figure 7.1

3. Gastric Surgery

Gastric surgery may cause malabsorption. The mechanisms are complex. Inadequate mixing of food with digestive juices in the stomach and rapid emptying of gastric contents into the small intestine are undoubtedly important factors. Uncoordinated release of pancreatic enzymes and bile into the small intestine leads to poor mixing with food and incomplete digestion. Bacterial contamination of the small bowel after a Polya type gastrectomy causes a *stagnant loop syndrome* (see below).

4. Bacterial colonization of small intestine

Colonization of the small intestine with large numbers of bacteria occurs after Polya gastrectomy and in other conditions which lead to stagnation or contamination of small bowel contents. These include small bowel diverticulosis, strictures and entero-colic fistulae, usually due to Crohn's disease, scleroderma and amyloidosis. Under these circumstances the *Bacteroides* group of organisms cause malabsorption of fat by interfering with bile salt metabolism in the lumen of the small intestine. *E. coli* utilize vitamin B_{12}, which may lead to a macrocytic anaemia.

5. Pancreatic insufficiency

Pancreatic insufficiency, usually due to chronic pancreatitis, causes malabsorption because there is a deficiency of enzymes to digest the large molecular constituents of food prior to absorption.

6. Hepatic and biliary disease

Hepatic and biliary disease may result in inadequate quantities of bile salts reaching the small intestine. It is very rare for hepatic or biliary disease to cause significant malabsorption in the absence of jaundice. Thus, this cause of malabsorption is easily identified and does not pose a diagnostic problem.

Commonest causes of malabsorption

The commonest causes of malabsorption in the UK are gastric surgery, coeliac disease, Crohn's disease and chronic pancreatitis. Less common are intestinal resection, small bowel lymphoma, chronic intestinal ischaemia, bowel damage due to radiotherapy, postinfective diarrhoea, giardiasis, tropical sprue and Whipple's disease.

Clinical features

Although the clinical picture may strongly suggest the aetiology, confirmatory investigation is necessary because specific management varies widely from one disorder to another. A patient with malabsorption will usually present with one or more of the following clinical features. The symptoms and signs are often individually unimpressive, but when they occur in combination the possibility of malabsorption should be seriously considered.

Diarrhoea and steatorrhoea

The severity of bowel disturbance varies widely and the absence of diarrhoea does not exclude the diagnosis of malabsorption. The pale, bulky, floating offensive stool said to be characteristic of malabsorption is also relatively rare. When the cause is Crohn's disease the stool may contain frank or occult blood. Identification of a fatty stool by inspection will point to the diagnosis of malabsorption and allow a more rational line of investigation to be planned.

Abdominal pain

Vague, poorly localized discomfort, accompanied by distension of the abdomen, is common. This symptom, however, has no discriminatory value as it is present in many gastrointestinal disorders. Chronic pancreatitis may cause a dull continuous pain in the upper abdomen with intermittent bouts of severe pain. This may radiate to the back and relief is sometimes obtained by leaning forward or lying prone. Colicky pain, in association with malabsorption, may be due to partial obstruction of the small bowel. This is most likely to be the result of Crohn's disease or, more rarely, lymphoma. In such patients an inflammatory or neoplastic mass is sometimes palpable.

Nutritional deficiencies

Nutritional deficiencies are rarely gross and may not be obvious on routine examination. However, mild deficiency of several different nutrients, either on clinical assessment or investigation, makes malabsorption a distinct possibility.

Constitutional disturbance   Some symptoms of malabsorption such as lethargy and lack of energy cannot be attributed to any particular nutritional disturbance. It is likely to be the result of multiple minor deficiencies and electrolyte depletion.

Weight loss   Weight loss is partly due to inadequate absorption of nutrients but in some diseases, such as Crohn's disease and lymphoma, anorexia is an important factor.

Anaemia   Tiredness, dyspnoea and, in the elderly, angina are common symptoms of anaemia. Because of the insidious onset of these symptoms they have often passed unnoticed and, in some patients, the anaemia is only brought to light by chance blood tests. In more severe cases, *angular stomatitis* and *glossitis* may be present.

Iron deficiency   The anaemia may be due to iron deficiency because of malabsorption from the upper small intestine in conditions such as coeliac disease or after gastrectomy. Iron deficiency in the latter may also be compounded by blood loss from the stomach due to gastritis or recurrent ulceration. Bleeding can also contribute to iron deficiency in Crohn's disease and small bowel lymphoma.

Folate and B_{12} deficiency   Macrocytic anaemia is caused by folate or vitamin B_{12} deficiency. Because folate is mainly absorbed in the upper small intestine, low levels are very common when the jejunum is the major site of pathology as in coeliac disease. In Crohn's disease, low folate levels are due to a combination of malabsorption, inadequate intake and increased metabolic utilization caused by the inflammatory nature of the disorder. Vitamin B_{12} is absorbed by the terminal ileum and, thus, longstanding disease or resection of this part of the intestine will inevitably give rise to deficiency. It is particularly common in Crohn's disease. Vitamin B_{12} malabsorption may also occur when there is *stasis in the small intestine*. This results because the proliferating bacteria metabolize the vitamin within the lumen of the bowel before it can be absorbed. The commonest causes of stasis and bacterial contamination of the small intestine are Polya gastrectomy, strictures and fistulae, usually due to Crohn's disease, and small bowel diverticulosis. A combined lack of iron and folate or vitamin B_{12} leads to a dimorphic blood film. This should always raise the suspicion of malabsorption and stimulate a search for its cause.

Anaemia is by far the commonest manifestation of nutritional deficiency due to malabsorption. The following deficiencies are very much rarer.

Osteomalacia and myopathy

Malabsorption of vitamin D may result in osteomalacia which often presents with limb pain. Weakness of girdle and proximal limb muscles, due to myopathy, is also found in a small number of patients. Serum calcium levels are frequently normal or only marginally lowered. The serum alkaline phosphatase is often raised. A minority have significantly reduced serum levels of calcium, and present with tetany.

Bruising

A slightly increased prothrombin time due to malabsorption of vitamin K may occur, but only very rarely is the deficiency severe enough to cause pathological bruising.

Oedema

Low serum albumin levels in malabsorption can occasionally be severe enough to cause oedema. This is partly caused by malabsorption of protein but in most cases it is the result of protein loss from a diseased small intestine. This condition is called *protein losing enteropathy*. It is most commonly due to coeliac disease, Crohn's disease and intestinal lymphoma. It should be remembered, however, that carcinomas of the stomach and large intestine and ulcerative colitis can also cause this disorder.

Neuropathy and psychiatric disorders

Peripheral neuropathy and disturbed mental function have been described in coeliac disease but both are rare. Surprisingly, there is no correlation with vitamin B_{12} deficiency and the aetiology remains unknown.

Other signs

Clubbing of the finger nails and *skin pigmentation*, in conjunction with the above features, though relatively rare, should increase the suspicion of small bowel disease. Patients with an irritant vesicular rash should be suspected of having *dermatitis herpetiformis*. Although these patients only rarely have clinical malabsorption, their nutritional status should be assessed by the simple haematological and biochemical tests outlined in the next section.

Special features

Apart from the presenting features, helpful information may be available from the past history. Previous *gastric or other abdominal surgery* is clearly important. *Abdominal or pelvic irradiation*, most commonly for carcinoma of the cervix, should be noted. A *history of diarrhoea and the use of special diets in childhood*, followed by normal health in adolescence without dietary treatment, is a common story in adults presenting with

86

coeliac disease. *Foreign travel*, particularly to south-east Asia and the Caribbean, raises the possibility of *tropical sprue* – even though these areas may not have been visited for many years. Infestation with *Giardia lamblia* is another possibility.

Alcohol abuse can cause diarrhoea and malabsorption of certain nutriments by a direct effect on the small intestine. It may also be associated with chronic pancreatitis and, in such patients, malabsorption is commonly accompanied by *recent onset of diabetes*. Conversely, as already discussed, *long-standing diabetes mellitus* can be complicated by diabetic diarrhoea due to changes in gut motility, bacterial flora and bile salt metabolism. *Scleroderma* involving the small intestine gives rise to malabsorption due to reduced motility and bacterial proliferation. The disease is invariably obvious from its cutaneous manifestations.

Investigation of suspected malabsorption

When malabsorption is suspected on clinical evidence, it is customary to back up the diagnosis with a small number of non-invasive investigations.

Serum iron, serum and red cell folate

In the British Isles, when the clinical suspicion of malabsorption is supported by *reduced blood levels of iron and folate* the most likely diagnosis is coeliac disease. It is, therefore now common practice to perform a small bowel biopsy

Small bowel biopsy

at this stage. This avoids unnecessary tests in the great majority of patients with malabsorption. Numerous capsules and tubes are available for obtaining small bowel biopsies but the most frequently used is the Crosby capsule or one of its modifications. The capsule and attached tube are swallowed and manoeuvred under radiological screening into the proximal jejunum. Alternatively, it may be passed in conjunction with a fibre optic endoscope. The latter methods makes rapid positioning of the capsule possible, and the entire procedure rarely takes more than 10 minutes. It is well tolerated and the incidence of complications is very low. In coeliac disease, the biopsy will characteristically reveal subtotal villous atrophy. Tropical sprue and the very rare conditions of Whipple's disease and intestinal lymphangiectasia can also be diagnosed by small bowel biopsy. The capsule almost invariably collects a small quantity of small bowel fluid which, in appropriate cases, should be examined microscopically for *Giardia lamblia* trophozoites.

When small bowel biopsy facilities are not readily avail-

Xylose absorption

able, or when the suspicion on clinical and haematological grounds is not so great, the *xylose absorption test* can provide helpful information. Xylose is a pentose which is readily absorbed from the small intestine. It is not metabolized in the body and is excreted unchanged in the urine. Both blood levels and the amount excreted in the urine after oral ingestion are measured. Used in this way the test will detect the great majority of patients with coeliac disease. This is because the diffuse lesion of the small intestine causes impaired absorption with resulting low blood and urine levels. By contrast, xylose absorption is usually normal in Crohn's disease in which the lesion is patchy or restricted to the terminal ileum. Similarly, in malabsorption due to pancreatic disease because the small intestine is normal, xylose absorption is unimpaired.

Antireticulin antibody

Another test that is useful in adding weight to the suspicion of coeliac disease is the antireticulin antibody test. It employs immunofluorescence to detect antibodies in the serum of patients with coeliac disease and is present in approximately 75% of untreated cases. *However, it must be emphasized that no other test can substitute for the small bowel biopsy in the diagnosis of coeliac disease.*

Radiology

If the small bowel biopsy is not diagnostic in patients suspected of having small bowel malabsorption, a barium follow-through examination is indicated. This will demonstrate those conditions that cause an anatomical abnormality. The commonest of these are Crohn's disease, lymphoma and small bowel diverticulosis. In patients with a history of gastric surgery or bowel resection it is often possible to assess the nature and extent of the operation. Fistulae between the large and small intestine may show on the follow-through but it is frequently necessary to perform a barium enema to demonstrate this type of abnormality. The so-called malabsorption pattern of the barium follow-through, which consists of an increase in the diameter of the lumen, thickened mucosal folds and flocculation of barium, can be found in malabsorption caused by both small intestinal and pancreatic disorders and is not diagnostic of any particular disease.

Faecal fat

When the above investigations have failed to provide a diagnosis, but malabsorption is still suspected, faecal fat estimation is indicated. A 5-day collection is necessary as there is wide daily variation of fat excretion. The test is delayed in the hope that it will not be required, because it usually necessitates admission to hospital and collection of stools is unpopular with patients, nurses and laboratory staff. Nevertheless, the demonstration that a patient excretes an average of more than 6 g of fat per day, whilst taking 70–100 g of fat in the diet, is good evidence of malabsorption and will encourage a continuing search for its cause.

Suspected pancreatic disease

If steatorrhoea is proved in the absence of previous stomach or intestinal surgery and small bowel radiology and biopsy are normal, the most likely cause is chronic pancreatitis.

The presence of diabetes mellitus or a diabetic *glucose tolerance test* and *calcification in the region of the pancreas* on abdominal X-ray reinforce the diagnosis. Reduced pancreatic function can be demonstrated in these cases. One test employs direct stimulation of the pancreas by injections of secretin and pancreozymin. Pancreatic juice is recovered, by intubation, from the duodenal lumen and the output and concentration of bicarbonate and enzymes are measured. The other commonly used investigation is the Lundh test. In this test the patient is given a standard homogenate of fat, carbohydrate and protein, via a tube positioned in the duodenum. This stimulates the secretion of pancreozymin and secretin from the duodenal mucosa which, in turn, induces pancreatic secretion. Duodenal fluid is aspirated and enzyme concentrations are measured.

Endoscopic retrograde pancreato-graphy

An alternative approach to confirming the diagnosis of chronic pancreatitis is by endoscopic retrograde pancreato-graphy. This investigation involves the passing of a fibre optic endoscope into the duodenum. A cannula is then passed via the biopsy channel of the endoscope and positioned in the ampulla of Vater. Radio contrast fluid is injected and X-ray films are taken of the pancreatic and biliary ducts. In chronic pancrea-titis the main and subsidiary ducts may be dilated, tortuous or strictured. Calculi and cysts may also be seen.

Suspected bacterial overgrowth

When the history or small bowel radiology points to the possibility of a stagnant loop syndrome, it can be confirmed by additional tests. The syndrome is caused by excessive numbers of colonic bacteria populating the small intestine. Quantitative culturing of small intestinal fluid is, therefore, the most direct and accurate method of confirming the diagnosis but it is not generally available.

Radioactive carbon bile salt breath test

The radioactive carbon bile salt breath test is more commonly used. In this test the patient takes orally a small quantity of conjugated bile salt, the amino acid of which is labelled with carbon 14. If there are excessive numbers of bacteria in the small intestine, the bile salt is deconjugated. This releases the labelled amino acid which is absorbed and metabolized in the body. The carbon of the amino acid is ultimately excreted in the breath as carbon dioxide. The amount of radioactivity in the breath can be measured and is proportional to the quantity of bile salt that was deconjugated which, in turn, reflects the degree of bacterial overgrowth. Although the 'radioactive breath test' is useful in the diagnosis of bacterial contamination of the small bowel, a positive result may also occur when the ileum is severely diseased or has been resected. This is because the labelled bile salt is not absorbed and passes into the colon. On entering the colon it is deconjugated and metabolized by large bowel bacteria, from where the radioactive label is absorbed. Thus, the test will not distinguish ileal disease or resection from small bowel bacterial overgrowth. However, by combining the result with the clinical and radiological features it is usually possible to decide which of these two mechanisms is operative.

Urinary indican The amino acid tryptophan is metabolized by bacteria in the small intestine to indole. This is absorbed and converted in the liver to indican, which is excreted in the urine. Excessive amounts suggest the possibility of a stagnant loop situation. It is not as accurate as bacterial culture of small bowel fluid or the radioactive bile salt breath test.

Vitamin B_{12} malabsorption Intrinsic factor is produced in the gastric mucosa and is essential for the specialized absorption of vitamin B_{12} from the terminal ileum. In pernicious anaemia, atrophy of the gastric glands leads to deficiency of intrinsic factor which, in turn, causes malabsorption of vitamin B_{12}. Malabsorption of vitamin B_{12} also occurs when the terminal ileum is diseased or has been resected. A third mechanism for the malabsorption of vitamin B_{12} is seen in small bowel stagnation. Under these circumstances the excessive numbers of bacteria, usually *E. coli*, metabolize the vitamin before it can be absorbed from the terminal ileum.

Schilling test The Schilling test is a means of measuring vitamin B_{12} absorption. A small amount of radioactively labelled B_{12} is taken orally, followed by a large intramuscular dose of non-labelled B_{12}. This causes vitamin B_{12}, including the labelled portion, to be flushed from the body. The amount of labelled B_{12} excreted in the urine over the next 24 h is proportional to the amount absorbed. If the test has been performed correctly and kidney function is normal, a low urinary excretion of radioactive label indicates malabsorption of vitamin B_{12}. In pernicious anaemia this can be corrected by the addition of exogenous intrinsic factor (part 2 Schilling test). This does not, of course, correct malabsorption of vitamin B_{12} when it is caused by disease or resection of the ileum or small bowel bacterial overgrowth. If bacterial overgrowth is the primary reason for malabsorption of vitamin B_{12}, it is frequently improved after a course of broad spectrum antibiotic therapy (part 3 Schilling test).

Protein losing enteropathy

When a protein losing enteropathy is suspected, it can be confirmed by the radioactive chromium 51 test. Radioactive chromium 51 is injected intravenously. This becomes attached to plasma albumin. If there is excessive loss of plasma protein into the gut due to diseases such as coeliac disease, Crohn's disease or lymphoma, large amounts of the radioactive label appear in the faeces.

Points to stress

- Diarrhoea and steatorrhoea are not always present in the malabsorption syndrome.
- Anaemia is the commonest presenting feature of small bowel malabsorption.

Problems with laxatives

Laxative abuse – Problems with specific laxatives

Laxative abuse

There are two main categories of laxative abusers.

Admitted long term users

Firstly, by far the larger group are those who present to the practitioner because they are concerned about an 'unsatisfactory' bowel habit and and the increasing amounts and variety of purgatives they need to take. There is usually a long history of taking laxatives, to which the patient will freely admit. Patients will complain that without laxatives no stool is passed for many days or weeks. Some resort to purgatives under these circumstances because with increasing constipation they experience abdominal pain and distension. Others wrongly attribute a multitude of symptoms, such as headaches and lethargy, to their sluggish bowel function. Some patients, however, have no accompanying symptoms but take laxatives as a habit because they firmly believe that a daily bowel movement is essential to health. This belief and ritual laxative usage has often started in childhood or adolescence. The majority have become dependent upon the chemical stimulant purgatives which include the anthraquinones (senna, cascara and danthron) or polyphenols (phenolphthalein and bisacodyl). Long term use of these drugs damages the myenteric plexus of the colon; this is probably the reason that increasing doses are required with chronic usage. The history of constipation, interspersed with bouts of passing poorly-formed stool, should always raise the possibility of large bowel cancer, even when the patient admits to recurrent use of laxatives. This is especially so in those over 40 years of age. Sigmoidoscopy and barium enema should, therefore, be performed. In purgative users, radiology will often reveal a featureless colon and in some there will be the characteristic smooth pseudostrictures of a cathartic colon. Sigmoidoscopy may show melanosis coli, which appears like dark freckles. They are due to lipofuschin contained in mucosal macrophages.

There are two main aims of management:

(1) To convince the patient that daily defaecation is not essential and that there is a wide variation of normal bowel function. Other symptoms such as lethergy, malaise and headache, which are attributed to constipation by the patient, should be treated on their merits. *They are often due to depression.*

(2) Attempts should also be made to re-educate the bowel. Following withdrawal of the stimulant laxative, it is almost invariably necessary to replace it initially with an osmotic purgative such as magnesium or sodium sulphate. Increasing dietary fibre with bran and products such as Normacol, Isogel and Metamucil are also important. The patient must be warned that it is likely to take several months for treatment to prove effective. Many will not persevere, and will return to their previous stimulant laxative abuse. In the elderly there is less chance of successful conversion to the new regime and it is often necessary for them to continue with stimulant laxatives.

In extremely rare cases the colon becomes totally unresponsive to increasing doses of purgative. Colectomy and ileorectal anastomosis may then be necessary.

Surreptitious abusers   The second category of laxative abusers are those who do so surreptitiously. They often present because of diarrhoea, but this may be denied. Other symptoms include abdominal discomfort and distension, thirst, lethargy and muscle weakness, due to dehydration and hypokalaemia. Less commonly steatorrhoea and protein losing enteropathy occur and clubbing, osteomalacia and oedema may also be present.

The patient is usually female and invariably psychologically disturbed. Many have coexistent anorexia nervosa and the abuse of other drugs, especially diuretics, is common. Denial of purgative usage hinders diagnosis and it is usually necessary to arrange hospital investigation to exclude other causes of metabolic disturbance. Such patients go to extraordinary lengths to conceal their actions. It may be necessary to search their lockers for purgatives and to test the stool for phenolphthalein and the urine for anthraquinone metabolites. Management is extremely difficult and depends mainly upon treatment of the underlying psychological disorders. Some authorities believe there is little to be gained by a confrontation with the patient. Such confrontation frequently results in her moving from one doctor to another or the precipitation of some other form of psychological disturbance.

Problems with specific laxatives

Liquid paraffin, which acts as a lubricant laxative, may – in large doses – impair absorption of the fat soluble vitamins, A, D and K. In old people it may seep through a lax anal sphincter causing soiling and pruritis ani. Aspiration pneumonitis, due to accidental inhalation, is another problem. It is particularly likely to occur in the elderly and debilitated or in the presence of oesophageal reflux, stricture or achalasia.

Surfactant laxatives such as dioctyl sodium sulphosuccinate and poloxalkol, which are constituents of Dulcodos and Dorbanex respectively, act by enhancing water penetration into stool. Recent evidence suggests they may interfere with small bowel absorption of concurrently taken drugs.

Osmotic laxatives are 'non-absorbable' compounds of sodium and magnesium. They are the major constituent of 'health salts'. By osmotic attraction they prevent absorption of water by the intestine which increases the fluidity of stool. Magnesium salts may also work by releasing cholecystokinin from the upper small intestine which, itself, affects colonic muscle activity. Overusage may cause electrolyte and fluid depletion. Although the majority of magnesium is not absorbed, small amounts do cross the intestinal mucosa. This is excreted in the urine but, in patients with renal impairment, hypermagnesaemia with muscle weakness and confusion may occur.

Bulk laxatives. These agents are non-absorbable, hydrophilic vegetable fibres. They stimulate bowel action mainly by virtue of their bulk and because they retain water the stool remains soft and manageable. They are the safest of the laxative preparations but should be avoided in patients with oesophageal or bowel strictures.

Stimulant laxatives (anthraquinones, polyphenols and castor oil). These drugs stimulate bowel peristalsis by direct action on the mucosa. They have a toxic effect on the myenteric plexus and may cause severe metabolic disturbance when used in excess over long periods.

Two drugs in this group cause specific problems. *Phenolphthalein* may induce skin irritation and rash which particularly affects the buttocks. *Oxyphenisatin* is contained in proprietary aperients available on the continent of Europe and in some preparations sold by 'health stores' in the United Kingdom. There is good evidence that it can cause a chronic active hepatitis.

Constipation and other problems with defaecation

Constipation – Other problems with defaecation

Constipation

It is important to realize that there is wide variation in the frequency of defaecation. Nevertheless, 90% of the population in the United Kingdom open their bowels between five times per week and twice per day. Only 1% has two or fewer bowel actions per week. Many of this latter group do not, however, have symptoms referable to constipation and doubtless accept their habit as normal. In contrast, there are many who quite naturally have a more frequent bowel action yet consider themselves constipated because they do not have a daily movement. This misconception often stems from childhood and the rigid attitude of parents to toilet training. Constipation is, therefore, difficult to define, but the term is probably best used to describe the *infrequent production of hard stool which requires excessive straining to pass.*

The great majority of patients presenting with constipation have no associated disease. This is termed *'simple' constipation.* Many have excessive segmenting movements of the colon which restrict the passage of stool and others appear to have reduced peristaltic movements. The mechanisms that control this smooth muscle activity are not understood. It seems likely that future research may reveal abnormalities of electrical activity and local neurotransmission. Whatever the mechanism, there is little doubt that lack of dietary fibre, inactivity and old age exacerbate the problem. Many patients with constipation have repeatedly *ignored the urge to defaecate* when the rectum is filled from the colon by peristalsis. This, in due course, leads to reduced sensitivity of the defaecating reflex. Increasing distension of the rectum is required to elicit the urge sensation, which is eventually lost. In such cases rectal examination frequently reveals a loaded rectum. In the majority of patients who deny this urge, the reasons are sociological rather than medical. These include embarrassment in requesting to leave classrooms and places of work and dislike of public lavatories. Other patients may have a painful local condition of the anus, such as fissure or piles and, therefore, try to pass stool as infrequently as possible.

There is an increased incidence of constipation in *pregnancy* but it is not clear whether this has a hormonal or mechanical basis. In a small minority of patients constipation may be a presenting or complicating feature of other disorders. Constipation is often a prominent symptom of the *irritable bowel syndrome.* The diagnosis is suggested by alternating diarrhoea and constipation, variable abdominal pain, the absence of blood loss per rectum and insignificant constitutional disturbance (p. 157).

Carcinoma of the left side of the colon or rectosigmoid junction may cause increasing constipation. The history is relatively short and there may be accompanying anorexia and weight loss. Blood may be noticed in the stool. Sigmoid tumours are often extrinsically palpable on rectal examination and visible with the sigmoidoscope. A double contrast barium enema will be necessary to exclude lesions beyond the range of the sigmoidoscope. *Strictures* resulting from *large bowel diverticulitis* and occasionally *colonic Crohn's disease* may also cause constipation. The history, barium enema and, when necessary, colonoscopy usually make the diagnosis clear.

Depression may often be accompanied by constipation but it is rarely the dominant presenting feature. *Hypothyroidism, hyperparathyroidism* and other causes of *hypercalcaemia* may cause constipation. Associated features of these disorders are almost invariably present.

It is essential to review *drug regimes* in those complaining of constipation. Antacids containing aluminium compounds and codeine-based cough linctuses are the commonest offenders. Other drugs less often implicated are anticholinergics and methyldopa.

Disease of the spinal cord or sacral nerve roots may cause constipation and rectal loading. There is nearly always accompanying bladder dysfunction, together with neurological symptoms and signs in the legs. *Hirschsprung's disease*, which is caused by an aganglionic segment in the distal bowel, is a cause of severe constipation and gross colonic distension in infants (see Problems in Paediatrics). A few, relatively mild cases, have apparently not presented until adult life but this must be extremely rare.

Management of simple constipation

Attention to those factors known to exacerbate constipation is often all that is needed. Patients should, therefore, be advised to increase the intake of fibre by including wholemeal bread, All-Bran or bran itself in their diet. Taking additional fluid and exercise will also help. It is most important that the patient is instructed to respond appropriately to the defaecation urge. He or she should also be reassured that a daily bowel action may not be normal for them and that there is no need to resort to potent laxatives if this is not achieved.

Special problems

Faecal impaction. Impaction of stool in the rectum or even sigmoid colon is the result of severe constipation. The main complaint may be of diarrhoea or incontinence due to seepage of fluid stool around the impacted mass. The problem is particularly likely to arise in the elderly, bedridden patients and paraplegics. A stool softening agent, such as the Dioctyl preparations, or olive oil as an enema should be used initially. These may be followed by stimulant laxatives such as Dulcolax and Senokot by mouth or glycerine or Dulcolax by suppository. If rectal loading persists, digital removal will be necessary. When the colon as well as rectum is loaded, sodium phosphate enemas are of value.

Maintenance regimes. Simple constipation will usually require no more treatment than previously discussed. Some patients will, nevertheless, require supplementary dietary fibre in order to maintain satisfactory bowel action. There are numerous preparations available, of which Fybogel, Normacol, Metamucil and Isogel are the most commonly used. Despite all of these measures, one is left with a small number of patients who require some additional help. It is not clear whether they are a specific subgroup who have an (as yet) undefined disturbance of colonic function. An osmotic purgative, such as lactulose, should be tried first but if this fails it may be necessary to allow the occasional use of stimulant laxatives, such as Senokot and Dulcolax.

Prophylaxis, when required, is as follows.

(1) Those undergoing surgery or other treatment for piles or fissure will need to keep their stools soft and thus avoid unnecessary pain. As this is a short term problem the choice of agent is not critical.

(2) It is wise to anticipate that enforced immobility, especially in the elderly, is likely to precipitate constipation. Preparations such as Milpar and lactulose are useful in these cases.

Other problems with defaecation

Alternating diarrhoea and constipation (see also p. 150).

The three main causes are the *irritable bowel syndrome, purgative abuse* and *carcinoma of the left colon* or *rectosigmoid junction*.

An erratic bowel habit is most commonly due to the irritable bowel syndrome. The history usually distinguishes it from laxative abuse, although purgation may be denied (p. 93).

Alternating diarrhoea and constipation of recent onset should always raise the suspicion of carcinoma in the left side of the colon or rectosigmoid junction. It is especially likely if there is accompanying weight loss, anorexia or blood loss per rectum. Sigmoidoscopy and barium enema are essential when these symptoms present.

Sensation of incomplete rectal emptying

Because *carcinoma of the rectum* often presents with this symptom, rectal examination and sigmoidoscopy are mandatory in such patients. Inflammatory conditions of the rectum, such as *ulcerative proctocolitis* and *Crohn's disease*, may also cause this sensation. The diagnosis is again made by sigmoidoscopy and rectal biopsy.

The *descending perineum syndrome* is characterized by a recurrent or continuous sensation of needing to defaecate. In this condition the anterior rectal mucosa prolapses, which causes a sensation of something in the lumen of the anus. Further straining only produces more prolapse. There is probably an underlying disorder of anorectal muscle function. Sigmoidoscopy will often reveal a small patch of 'proctitis' on the anterior rectal wall in the vicinity of the rectal valve. Treatment consists of explanation and reassurance. The patient must be discouraged from straining and any coexistent constipation must be treated.

Solitary ulcer of the anterior rectum appears to be a long term complication of the descending perineum syndrome. Patients with this condition are often obsessed by their bowel habit and frequently admit to digitally removing stool from the rectum. Sigmoidoscopy and biopsy distinguishes the ulcer from cancer. Treatment is unsatisfactory. When conservative measures fail some surgeons will attempt correction of the underlying prolapse.

The sensation of incomplete emptying may also occur in association with other symptoms in the *irritable bowel syndrome*. The usual complaint is that within minutes of passing stool the sensation to defaecate returns. Attempts to do so, however, result only in the passage of a few tiny pellet or thread-like stools. Increasing the bulk of the stool with additional dietary fibre is often very helpful.

Proctalgia fugax

This term is used to describe sudden severe pain in the perineum and rectum. It may occur spontaneously, or be precipitated by straining at stool and sexual intercourse. Nocturnal attacks are not uncommon. It lasts only a few seconds or minutes. The mechanism is not clear but probably results from spasm in the muscles of the pelvic floor or rectum. In those patients whose symptoms are brought on by straining at stool treatment includes relief of constipation. Pressure over the coccyx sometimes helps during an attack but there is otherwise no specific therapy. In patients experiencing frequent nocturnal attacks, or in those where sexual intercourse commonly precipitates the problem, diazepam is sometimes a useful prophylaxis. With reassurance most patients are able to tolerate their symptoms because the episodes are both infrequent and brief.

Point to stress

- Recent onset of constipation in patients over 40 requires early investigation by sigmoidoscopy and barium enema to exclude colorectal cancer.

10 Gastrointestinal bleeding

Acute upper gastrointestinal haemorrhage – Chronic or recurrent bleeding – Rectal bleeding

Bleeding from the gastrointestinal tract may be acute or chronic. *Acute haemorrhage* from the oesophagus, stomach and upper small intestine gives rise to haematemesis and/or melaena, whereas bleeding from the lower small intestine and caecum results in melaena alone. Patients bleeding from sites distal to the ascending colon pass identifiable blood per rectum. *Chronic bleeding* from the alimentary tract frequently causes no noticeable change in the faeces and the commonest presentation is anaemia.

Acute upper gastrointestinal haemorrhage

Common causes

In Britain, bleeding from the upper gastrointestinal tract accounts for approximately 25 000 admissions to hospital each year. The mortality is between 5 and 10%. The commonest causes are duodenal ulcer (40%), gastric ulcer (15%) and gastric erosions (15%). Oesophagitis, gastric cancer and tears of the lower oesophagus each constitute 5%. *Bleeding* due to oesophageal varices is rare in Britain and accounts for only 3% of patients presenting to district general hospitals. The percentage figures are approximate and are derived from several studies completed during the past 25 years. Other gastric tumours, such as leiomyomas and acute 'stress' ulcers following burns and shock, are also relatively rare causes. Despite the widespread use of endoscopy, no definite cause is established in about 10% of patients.

103

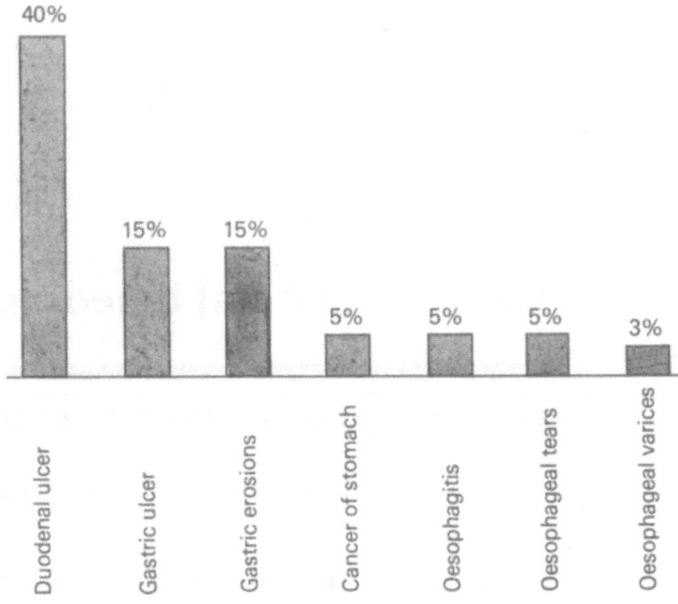

Causes of upper gastrointestinal bleeding in the UK (cumulative figures 1955–80)

Figure 10.1

Assessment of severity

Most patients who have a haematemesis are in no doubt that the blood was vomited. However, blood discovered in the mouth may have originated from the postnasal space or lower respiratory tract. This can cause confusion unless time is taken to elicit an accurate history. The haematemesis may consist either of fresh blood mixed with gastric fluid or changed blood in the form of 'coffee grounds'. *All such patients should be referred to hospital for admission because haematemesis indicates a recent haemorrhage.*

The patient's estimate of how much blood has been vomited is seldom helpful in assessing the true severity of the bleed. In contrast, vomitus saved by the patient or produced in the presence of the practitioner is a useful guide. Haematemesis may be accompanied by melaena but because most patients who vomit blood rapidly seek medical attention, it is not always initially present. If no stool has been passed, rectal examination may reveal melaena. This can sometimes be helpful when there is doubt about the validity of haematemesis. Melaena without haematemesis often indicates a less severe bleed. However, *when melaena is fresh or has been present for 3 days or less, admission to hospital is still required.* A patient with a longer history of melaena who is not anaemic and remains otherwise healthy does not necessarily require admission, providing early investigation can be arranged. Confusion can sometimes arise in patients taking iron or bismuth containing preparations because they both cause darkening of the stool. Neither gives a positive occult blood test.

Physical signs following gastrointestinal haemorrhage are misleading and frequently underestimate the true blood loss. Pallor of the skin, a pulse rate of greater than 100/min and a systolic blood pressure of less than 100 mmHg or a diastolic pressure of less than 65 mmHg, indicate the need for blood transfusion. These measurements taken with the patient lying down may not always detect hypovolaemia. Thus, if normal, they should be repeated with the patient sitting or standing. A drop in pressure and rise in pulse rate are indications of a significant reduction in blood volume. Estimation of the central venous pressure is an even more accurate means of assessing the degree of hypovolaemia. A haemoglobin concentration of less than 9 g/100 ml suggests severe haemorrhage. However, normal levels do not exclude this, because vasoconstriction can maintain a misleadingly high haemoglobin concentration.

Initial management

In most hospitals patients with haematemesis and melaena are admitted under the care of a physician. However, because surgery plays an important part in the management of many patients, the surgical team should be advised of the admission and kept closely informed about the patient's progress.

Blood transfusion

As previously discussed, blood transfusion will be required for *all* patients who have clear evidence of a significant bleed, indicated by a large substantiated haematemesis, fluid melaena, anaemia or low arterial and central venous pressures. In such patients a minimum of 4 units is usually required to replace the loss. If more than 6 units are needed, 10 ml of 10% calcium gluconate should be given to restore serum calcium levels. Whilst awaiting cross-matched blood, the blood volume can be partially restored with either plasma or synthetic macromolecular infusion fluids. This preliminary measure is particularly important when shock is evident. In patients who, on clinical grounds, appear to have suffered a less severe bleed, an infusion should be set up and maintained with normal saline or dextrose. Blood should be cross-matched and kept in readiness. As with all patients after haematemesis and melaena the pulse and blood pressure are measured at least hourly. If these estimations indicate continued bleeding or the patient produces fresh haematemesis or melaena, blood should be given without further delay. In many centres, central venous pressure is recorded in conjunction with pulse and arterial pressure because it provides earlier evidence of further bleeding and enables the blood volume to be restored more accurately. In patients with shock, metabolic acidosis can be corrected with an infusion of sodium bicarbonate.

Oral fluids and food   Oral fluids should be encouraged from the start and food taken if the patient feels hungry.

Drugs   Anxiety is best allayed by the prompt institution of the measures already mentioned and strong reassurance. A small dose of diazepam may also be helpful. Antacids or cimetidine should be given for dyspeptic pain but, as yet, there is no clear evidence that either arrests haemorrhage or prevents rebleeding from peptic ulcers.

The site of bleeding   *In gastrointestinal haemorrhage, establishing the cause of bleeding is secondary to assessment of severity and resuscitation.*

Clinical features   Although a previous peptic ulcer history may be helpful, it does not prove that there is an existing ulcer or that it is the site of haemorrhage. Furthermore, a significant proportion of patients who bleed from peptic ulcers have no history of dyspepsia. Aspirin and anti-inflammatory drugs cause gastrointestinal haemorrhage. However, the role of aspirin in clinically apparent gastrointestinal haemorrhage has probably been overstated. A history of aspirin consumption during the previous 48 h does not necessarily indicate that bleeding is due to gastric erosions. The evidence that steroids cause significant gastrointestinal haemorrhage is even more tenuous. Alcohol abuse may be a factor in patients with peptic ulcer, gastric erosions, varices or oesophageal tears. In the latter, which are not always alcohol induced, haematemesis is usually preceded by an initial vomit that produces no blood.

Although cutaneous signs of chronic liver disease, ascites and splenomegaly suggest the possibility of variceal bleeding, it should be remembered that peptic ulcer and gastric erosions are also commonly associated with cirrhosis. A history or signs of recent weight loss, anorexia, or a mass in the epigastrium points to a diagnosis of stomach cancer. Carcinoma of the caecum may give rise to melaena. A palpable mass in the right iliac fossa and a change in bowel habit are other features of this disease.

The great majority of patients with gastrointestinal haemorrhage have a local lesion in the gut. Nevertheless, in a small proportion more generalized disease is responsible. Such diseases include bleeding diatheses, leukaemia, polyarteritis nodosa, Henoch–Schönlein purpura and chronic renal failure. Other features of these disorders are usually present or obvious after simple routine investigations.

Investigation In most hospitals the quickest means of identifying the cause of bleeding is endoscopy. An accurate diagnosis can be obtained in 90% of cases. Similar success can be achieved in some centres with a double contrast barium meal. At present there is no clearcut evidence that routine emergency endoscopy or barium meal plays an important part in early management. Many hospitals have, nevertheless, adopted a policy of 'early' endoscopy which usually means that the examination is performed within 24–36 h of admission. Although this policy has yet to make any impact on mortality, it makes an earlier discharge from hospital possible and may, in the future, lead to reduced morbidity and mortality. When endoscopy of the upper gastrointestinal tract has failed to find the cause of melaena, carcinoma of the caecum must be considered. In the majority, double contrast barium enema will confirm the diagnosis but, if doubt remains, colonoscopy may be necessary.

Further management The majority of patients have a single episode of bleeding which ceases within 24 h. Such cases are readily managed by the medical measures already discussed. Future elective treatment will clearly depend upon the nature of the underlying lesion. Unfortunately, a considerable number continue to haemorrhage or rebleed. It is in this group that the great majority of fatalities occur. The factors particularly associated with recurrent bleeding are a presenting haematemesis, chronic gastric ulcer and oesophageal varices. Vigilance and intensive observation, as previously outlined, are vital during the first 48 h because approximately 90% of all rebleeding occurs during this period.

Patients under the age of 50 tolerate rebleeding and further blood transfusion relatively well. In this group it is, therefore, usual to persevere with conservative management. Even so, some of these patients will require emergency surgery because of continuing haemorrhage.

Surgery Over the age of 50 recurrent bleeding and need for continuing transfusion are accompanied by a greatly increased mortality. Early surgical intervention is therefore favoured. By the time the patient comes to surgery, the site of bleeding will usually have been identified by endoscopy. Most patients requiring surgery are bleeding from a vessel in the floor of a peptic ulcer and haemorrhage is stopped by a simple suture procedure. In the elderly and severely ill this may be the only procedure undertaken. However, in some patients it will also be possible to perform more definitive surgery, such as resection of a gastric ulcer or, in those with duodenal ulcer, vagotomy and pyloroplasty. Gastric erosions and oesophageal tears can usually be managed conservatively, although surgery will be required if haemorrhage continues.

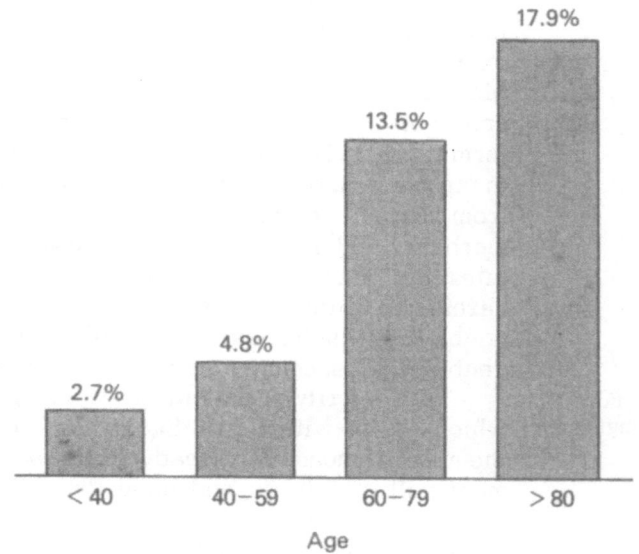

Age

Effect of age on death rate in patients admitted to Radcliffe Infirmary, Oxford with haematemesis and melaena

Figure 10.2

Endoscopic
photo-
coagulation

Photocoagulation of bleeding points with a laser beam under endoscopic control is a probable future development.

Bleeding from
oesophageal
varices

At present oesophageal varices are a relatively rare cause of gastrointestinal bleeding in the United Kingdom. It is likely to become a more common cause, given the increasing incidence of alcoholic cirrhosis. Diagnostic and general resuscitative procedures have already been discussed, but with variceal haemorrhage there are additional problems. Bleeding in chronic liver disease often precipitates hepatic encephalopathy. This is characterized by a variable reduction in intellectual performance and consciousness which is accompanied by a flapping tremor and foetor. Encephalopathy improves with cessation of bleeding but additional prompt attention must be given to correction of electrolyte imbalance and treatment of coexistent infection. The colon must be washed out. Magnesium sulphate, lactulose and neomycin should be given by mouth or nasogastric tube to reduce production and absorption of toxic colonic bacterial metabolites.

Continuing haemorrhage

Vasopressin

Bleeding from varices frequently fails to stop spontaneously. When haemorrhage continues, intravenous vasopressin should be given. This can be administered as bolus injections of 20 units in 100 ml of 5% dextrose or as an infusion at the rate of 0.4 units/min for up to 24 h. Vasopressin frequently stops bleeding but recurrence is very common when it is withdrawn. Nevertheless, it buys time during which further information can be obtained and other forms of treatment organized. Side-effects include abdominal pain, evacuation of the bowels and constriction of coronary arteries. It should, therefore, be used with extreme caution in patients suffering from ischaemic heart disease.

Balloon compression

Local compression of varices with a Sengstaken tube is another means of arresting haemorrhage. Modern versions of this tube incorporate balloons that can be inflated in the stomach and oesophagus to compress the bleeding varices. It also includes tubes through which secretions from the stomach and proximal oesophagus can be aspirated. The use of these tubes for 24–48 h aids resuscitation and allows time for more definitive measures to be planned. Bleeding in patients with liver disease is likely to be complicated by a deficiency of clotting factors and thrombocytopenia. Fresh plasma and platelet infusion may, therefore, be necessary.

Surgery

If bleeding recurs when the Sengstaken tube is deflated surgery is usually necessary. In the emergency situation this most frequently consists of simple ligation of the varices or oesophageal transection and re-anastomosis. The alternative is to construct a shunt anastomosis between the portal and systemic venous systems. These procedures lower the flow through the varices, thus reducing the tendency to haemorrhage. Performed as an emergency, shunt operations have an extremely high mortality. It is, therefore, current practice to stop haemorrhage by simpler measures and to consider shunting only as an elective procedure. Prior to an elective shunt it is necessary to obtain more information about the site of obstruction and size and patency of the veins that are to be anastomosed. The most commonly used techniques are splenic venography, mesenteric arteriography and ultrasound. A successful outcome following a shunt operation is adversely affected by previous persistent encephalopathy, jaundice, hypo-albuminaemia and ascites. The major problems after operation are a worsening of hepatic function and encephalopathy. The best results are achieved in patients with extrahepatic obstruction of the portal venous system and the worst in those with intrahepatic obstruction due to advanced cirrhosis.

Sclerosant therapy   In recent years, injection of oesophageal varices with sclerosant fluid via an endoscope has been advocated as a means of preventing haemorrhage. More information is required before the procedure's true efficacy can be assessed, but it is likely that it will reduce the need for shunt operations in a large number of patients.

Chronic or recurrent bleeding

. Recurrent haematemesis is relatively uncommon because vomiting blood usually follows a severe bleed which demands urgent attention. Furthermore, as the bleeding has come from the oesophagus, stomach or duodenum, endoscopic diagnosis can be readily made and early definitive treatment given. The exception to this is the patient with varices who may have several haematemeses before a decision is made about future management policy.

In contrast, chronic or recurrent loss of smaller amounts of blood from the oesophagus, stomach, small intestine and caecum most commonly presents as *iron deficiency anaemia* and more rarely as *melaena*. Haemorrhage from more distal sites usually appears as identifiable blood *per rectum* and is discussed below (Rectal bleeding). All the conditions that commonly cause acute bleeding may present with chronic blood loss. Attention to the previously discussed clinical features, together with endoscopy and appropriate barium studies, will reveal the site of bleeding in the majority of cases. When melaena is not obvious, alimentary tract bleeding can be confirmed by examination of stools for occult blood.

The following are less common causes of chronic gastro-intestinal bleeding.

(1) *Hereditary haemorrhage telangiectasia* in which the char-acteristic lesions can be seen on the lips and buccal mucosa,

around the nostrils and beneath the nails. The mode of inheritance is autosomal dominance and a family history of the condition can usually be obtained.

(2) *Lymphoma* of the gut must always be suspected when routine investigation has failed to demonstrate the cause of bleeding. Diarrhoea, constitutional disturbance, abdominal masses, peripheral lymphadenopathy and splenomegaly may also be present.

(3) *Polyposis* of the small intestine is a rare cause of recurrent blood loss. In the Peutz–Jeghers syndrome, hamartomatous polyps are associated with dark brown pigmentation of the lips and buccal mucosa. A family history is usual because the condition is inherited as an autosomal dominant. A barium follow-through examination confirms these two latter disorders.

(4) Residence in the developing countries of the world should raise the possibility of infestation, particularly with *hookworm*. Stool examination is diagnostic.

(5) In patients who have artificial intra-abdominal *arterial grafts*, recurrent melaena may indicate a fistula between gut and artery. The commonest site is between the aorta and third part of the duodenum. It is important to be aware of this possibility, as relatively small bleeds often precede a massive fatal haemorrhage.

Angiography   When barium studies and endoscopy have failed to demonstrate the site of bleeding, *angiography* should be considered. If selective arteriography of mesenteric arteries is performed during an episode of bleeding it is often possible to see extravasation of the radio-opaque medium from the lesion. Even when it is not possible to study the patient at the time of bleeding, arteriography may show the typical pattern of a vascular *tumour* or *angiodysplasia*.

Points to stress

- Haematemesis indicates recent haemorrhage and the need for hospital admission.
- In a patient with gastrointestinal bleeding, a postural drop in blood pressure and rise in pulse rate indicates hypovolaemia and need for urgent blood replacement.
- A normal haemoglobin does not exclude significant blood loss.

111

Rectal bleeding

Rectal bleeding means the passage of identifiable blood per rectum, as distinct from melaena stool. The symptom is usually the result of blood loss from the rectum or colon but brisk bleeding from the upper gastrointestinal tract can occasionally give rise to unchanged blood being passed per rectum. However, rectal bleeding is rarely massive and, unlike haematemesis and melaena, urgent hospital admission is only occasionally required.

Investigations   As discussed below the history and full examination provide valuable clues to the likely cause which reduces the chance of unnecessary investigation. It is clearly impractical for every patient who notices small amounts of blood on the toilet paper or stool to be extensively investigated, but *digital examination and sigmoidoscopy are obligatory*. If a local anal lesion seems to be the probable cause appropriate treatment should be given. If, despite this, bleeding continues or no obvious cause is found, or there is suspicion on clinical evidence of a more proximal lesion then *a double contrast barium enema or colonoscopy is indicated*. In those cases which still defy diagnosis *arteriography*, especially during the bleeding phase, is frequently valuable. *Laparotomy* to identify the source of rectal bleeding is often unrewarding and is now only employed when other investigations have failed or life is threatened by massive bleeding.

Common causes

Haemorrhoids   The commonest cause of rectal blood loss is *haemorrhoids* and they account for approximately 90 per cent of cases with this presenting symptom. Blood may be noticed both on the paper and coating the stool. On other occasions straining at stool may result in fresh blood being passed alone. In the absence of thrombosis there is little pain. Third degree haemorrhoids are obvious to both the patient and doctor. Second degree piles are confirmed by asking the patient to strain. First degree piles are verified by proctoscopy.

First and minor second degree piles are best treated by injection of a sclerosant. Larger second degree and third degree disease requires either haemorrhoidectomy or manual dilatation under anaesthesia. Because patients have often suffered with longstanding constipation the opportunity must also be taken to regulate the bowel habit, preferably with bulk laxatives, in order to reduce the chance of recurrence.

Anal fissure

Although an anal fissure often causes bleeding the predominant symptom in most patients is *pain on defaecation.* Diagnosis is confirmed by gently parting the buttocks. Most fissures occur posteriorly. It is often impossible to perform further examination of the rectum at presentation. Many cases respond to regular use of an anal dilator after digital application of an anaesthetic gel. Proctoscopy should be undertaken when it becomes possible to do so in order to exclude additional pathology such as inflammatory bowel disease or carcinoma. More severe cases and those that do not respond to dilatation will require partial surgical division of the internal anal sphincter.

Polyps

In the absence of local anal disease, polyps of the large bowel are probably the commonest cause of rectal bleeding. *It is usually the only symptom.* Diagnosis is made by sigmoidoscopy and *double contrast* barium enema. *A single contrast barium study will miss the majority of small polyps.* It may be necessary to proceed to diagnostic colonoscopy when these investigations are unfruitful. The colonoscope also provides a means of resecting the lesions without need of laparotomy and colotomy. It is now accepted practice to remove all adenomatous polyps because there is good evidence that some progress to carcinoma.

Large bowel cancer

The majority of colorectal carcinomas bleed but this is often occult or slight. Severe bleeding is rare. Rectal bleeding may be the only symptom but associated complaints are an altered bowel habit, abdominal pain and tenesmus. Anorexia and weight loss, though often present, are not as common as in many other malignant diseases. Examination may reveal anaemia or an abdominal mass. Digital examination of the rectum will demonstrate a high proportion of rectal cancers and many in the sigmoid colon will also be palpable extrinsically. Investigations are the same as those used for the diagnosis of large bowel polyps. *Sixty per cent of all large bowel cancers can be diagnosed by sigmoidoscopy.*

Inflammatory bowel disease

Both Crohn's disease and ulcerative colitis may present with rectal bleeding but in both conditions *it is usually accompanied by diarrhoea* and in Crohn's disease by *abdominal pain.* An histological diagnosis is made by sigmoidoscopic or colonoscopic biopsy. The extent of the disease is defined either by double contrast barium enema or colonoscopy.

Diverticular disease

In developed countries diverticula of the colon occur in more than a third of the population over 60. They are, therefore, seen commonly on barium enema in patients being investigated for rectal bleeding. Although there is no doubt that colonic diverticula bleed either occultly or overtly, their presence should not dissuade the practitioner from continued observation or investigation of the patient if there is suspicion of an alternative pathology. Angiography during a phase of bleeding is the best means of confirming that blood loss is arising from a diverticulum.

Rarer causes

Infection   Both amoebic and *Shigella* dysentery cause rectal bleeding but both are very rarely seen in the British Isles.

Salmonella and *Campylobacter* may affect the large intestine but bleeding is always accompanied by diarrhoea and the illness is shortlived.

Ischaemia   Ischaemia of the colon may lead to bleeding per rectum. Associated features are pain, guarding, pyrexia and systemic disturbance. It is commonest in the elderly and there is usually other evidence of cardiovascular disease. The ischaemia may cause infarction of large areas of the colon, requiring resection. Alternatively, there may be complete resolution with return of normal bowel function within a few days. Some patients develop ischaemic strictures which cause obstructive symptoms. Many of these resolve spontaneously over a period of weeks or months but some require surgical resection.

Angio-   Angiodysplasia is a recently recognized vascular abnor-
dysplasia   mality of gut mucosa which may give rise to either melaena or recognizable blood per rectum. It is most common in elderly patients and is probably a degenerative disorder. The right colon is the usual site. The lesion consists of abnormal superficial vessels in the mucosa which can best be demonstrated by angiography. The condition can also be found at colonoscopy by which means it may also be possible to cauterize localized areas of disease. When the lesion is more extensive colonic resection is often necessary.

Massive rectal bleeding

As previously mentioned, massive rectal bleeding is an uncommon event. The causes in adults are: diverticular disease, inflammatory bowel disease, colorectal tumours and angiodysplasia. A Meckel's diverticulum should also be considered in adolescents and young adults.

Admission to hospital is always necessary. The management is essentially similar to that for upper gastrointestinal haemorrhage with resuscitative measures taking precedence over diagnostic procedures. Investigations are those described previously. Endoscopic examinations are frequently obscured by blood and for this reason angiography, if available, is often preferred. A vasopressin infusion may temporarily stop bleeding, thus giving more time for the organization of treatment and investigation.

11 Diagnosis of the common causes of jaundice

Unconjugated hyperbilirubinaemia – Hepatocellular and cholestatic jaundice

Serum bilirubin in jaundice

Pathophysiological classification

Jaundice occurs when the total bilirubin level in the serum rises above 2 mg per 100 ml or 17 μmol/l. On a pathophysiological basis jaundice can be classified under the following headings:

haemolysis,
dyserythropoiesis,
non-haemolytic hyperbilirubinaemias,
hepatocellular,
extra- and intrahepatic cholestasis.

Although this facilitates an understanding of the mechanisms involved it has no particular merit in the everyday clinical situation. When faced with a jaundiced patient it is simpler to consider the common causes of jaundice and by careful analysis of clinical, haematological, biochemical and imaging data the diagnosis can be achieved rapidly in most instances. An early decision can then be made regarding the need for surgery or the adoption of medical management.

Unconjugated hyperbilirubinaemia

Haemolytic disease, dyserythropoiesis, the commonest cause of which is pernicious anaemia, and the non-haemolytic unconjugated hyperbilirubinaemias are characterized by raised levels of unconjugated bilirubin in the serum. Unconjugated bilirubin is not passed in the urine and, therefore, in contrast to hepatocellular and cholestatic disease, bilirubinuria is not found in these disorders.

Haemolytic disease and dyserythro-poiesis

Jaundice occurs in haemolytic and dyserythropoietic disease when the liver is presented with an excess of haem metabolites which swamp the conjugating process.

Because jaundice is a relatively minor feature of adult haemolytic disease and dyserythropoiesis it is rarely a presenting symptom in these conditions. They are readily distinguished from hepatocellular and cholestatic disease because of the accompanying anaemia, reticulocytosis, appearances of the blood film and bone marrow and absence of bile in the urine.

Gilbert's disease

Gilbert's disease is the only commonly encountered cause of non-haemolytic unconjugated hyperbilirubinaemia. The mode of inheritance is probably autosomal dominance. Jaundice is due to a deficiency of the hepatic enzyme UDP glucuronyl transferase which is necessary for the efficient conversion of unconjugated bilirubin to the conjugated form. It is only the conjugated form that can be excreted in bile and therefore the levels of unconjugated bilirubin rise in the serum. A significant deficiency of the enzyme is present in approximately 5% of the British population, but clinically apparent icterus from this disorder is rare. Jaundice can be precipitated or exacerbated in Gilbert's disease by starvation. Anorexia induced by any illness may, therefore, be accompanied by mild jaundice in those with Gilbert's disease. As a consequence there is sometimes confusion with viral hepatitis. The two conditions are easily distinguished because in Gilbert's disease the serum alkaline phosphatase and transaminase levels are normal and there is no bile in the urine.

Clinical distinction from viral hepatitis

Hepatocellular and cholestatic jaundice

The great majority of patients presenting with jaundice have either hepatocellular or cholestatic disease. The common causes and the predominant mechanism for jaundice are shown in Table 11.1.

Clinical features in hepatocellular and cholestatic jaundice

Anorexia

Weight loss

Anorexia and nausea for a few days prior to the appearance of jaundice is characteristic of viral hepatitis. Reduction of appetite over a longer period accompanied by weight loss suggests malignant disease.

118

Table 11.1   Common causes of jaundice in the British Isles

Cause	Main mechanism
Viral hepatitis	Hepatocellular
Alcoholic hepatitis	Hepatocellular
Drugs	Hepatocellular or intrahepatic cholestasis
Gallstones	Extrahepatic cholestasis
Carcinoma of pancreas	Extrahepatic cholestasis
Secondary hepatic carcinoma	Intrahepatic and extrahepatic cholestasis
Chronic hepatitis	Hepatocellular
Primary biliary cirrhosis	Intrahepatic cholestasis
Cirrhosis alcoholic autoimmune hepatitis B cryptogenic	Hepatocellular and intrahepatic cholestasis

Malaise

General ill health, often with recurrent bouts of jaundice over many months is frequently found in cirrhosis or chronic active hepatitis.

Colitis

Ulcerative colitis may be complicated by chronic liver disease and in a few patients the bowel disease will not have been previously diagnosed.

Dark urine and pale stool

Bilirubinuria and a decrease in biliary pigment in the stool may result from widespread hepatocellular disease, as in hepatitis, or obstruction of the biliary system by any mechanism.

Pyrexia

Patients with viral hepatitis usually have only a modest fever. By contrast bacterial cholangitis, which is generally the result of cholelithiasis or stricture of the common bile duct, is characterized by a high swingeing fever. Chills and rigors commonly accompany the pyrexia. Septicaemia from any source may occasionally sufficiently disturb hepatic function to cause jaundice.

Chills and rigors

Pain

Severe epigastric pain which often radiates to the shoulder region strongly suggests biliary colic. There may have been several episodes of the same pain not accompanied by jaundice during the previous months or years. A continuous boring pain in the upper abdomen radiating to the back and eased by leaning forward is typical of carcinoma of the pancreas. Both viral and alcoholic hepatitis can cause pain in the right hypochondrium which varies greatly in severity from one patient to another.

Itching

Pruritis is due to retention of bile salts in the blood. It is most frequently found in diseases that cause obstruction to the biliary system such as cholelithiasis, carcinoma of the pancreas, phenothiazine jaundice and primary biliary cirrhosis. In the latter it often precedes jaundice by many months or years. However, pruritis is sometimes a feature of acute viral hepatitis.

Rash
Arthritis

Jaundice caused by type B hepatitis and glandular fever is often accompanied by a rash. Arthritis is also common in type B virus disease, whereas lymphadenopathy and sore throat is suggestive of glandular fever.

Drugs

An accurate and detailed drug history from the patient, relatives and other practitioners is vital. Herbal preparations should be noted, especially any that contain the laxative oxyphenisatin. Halothane jaundice should be considered in any patient who has recently undergone surgery.

Alcohol

Both past and present drinking habits must be ascertained. A binge may precipitate an attack of acute alcoholic hepatitis in a patient with well compensated cirrhosis who had not been previously jaundiced.

Surgery

A past history of cholecystectomy especially when this has been preceded or accompanied by jaundice should raise the suspicion of a retained gallstone or bile duct stricture.

Chemical
exposure

Many aromatic chemicals, especially the chlorinated forms are hepatotoxic and a history of exposure is clearly relevant in the investigation of jaundice.

Blood
products

Screening of blood for hepatitis virus type B has reduced the chances of contracting viral hepatitis from blood transfusion. But other viruses especially the non-A, non-B virus may still be transmitted in this way.

Contaminated
needles

Ineffective sterilization of tattooists' instruments and communal use of syringes and needles by drug addicts are other means of transmitting viral hepatitis.

Male
homosexuals

Hepatitis viruses especially type B may be venereally transmitted and this is a particular problem in male homosexuals.

Oedema and
ascites

Jaundice accompanied by oedema is most likely to be due to cirrhosis. Ascites is common in cirrhosis but may also occur in the patient whose jaundice is due to secondary hepatic carcinoma. Rarely jaundice may be seen in a patient with ascites and oedema due to severe congestive cardiac failure.

Cutaneous
signs

The finding of cutaneous signs, such as white nails, clubbing, bruising, loss of body hair, spider naevi and palmar erythema suggest cirrhosis or chronic active hepatitis. In acute hepatitis spider naevi and palmar erythema may transiently appear.

Xanthelasma

Cutaneous lipid deposits may accompany *longstanding*

cholestasis which in most cases is due to primary biliary cirrhosis.

Gynaecomastia
Testicular atrophy
Hypertrophy of breast tissue in men and testicular atrophy are most commonly seen in cirrhosis but also occur in chronic active hepatitis and alcoholic hepatitis.

Parotid enlargement and Dupuytren's contractures
Dupuytren's contractures and hypertrophy of the parotid salivary glands should raise the suspicion of alcohol-related disease.

Lymphadenopathy
Enlarged lymph nodes in the neck or supraclavicular fossae are most likely to be due to metastases from a lung or intra-abdominal carcinoma. More rarely lymphoma may be the cause of lymphadenopathy and jaundice.

Hepatomegaly
A large smooth-edged liver is commonly found in alcoholic liver disease. Tenderness suggests hepatitis and this may be severe in acute alcoholic hepatitis. A hard irregular edge to the liver is most likely to be due to secondary carcinoma but also occurs in macronodular cirrhosis.

Palpable gall bladder
A palpable gall bladder is usually indicative of extra-hepatic obstruction of the biliary system and usually the result of pancreatic cancer.

Splenomegaly
Dilated abdominal veins and splenomegaly are the hallmarks of portal hypertension. When associated with jaundice they are almost always due to cirrhosis or chronic active hepatitis.

Investigation of hepatocellular and cholestatic jaundice (see Figure 11.1)

Standard liver function tests are of limited value in diagnosing the cause of jaundice.

Serum bilirubin
The highest levels of bilirubin in plasma tend to occur when the biliary system is obstructed as in carcinoma of the pancreas. A steadily increasing concentration of bilirubin is highly suggestive of this diagnosis. In hepatitis and chronic liver disease the levels are variable.

Alkaline phosphatase
Very high levels of alkaline phosphatase (over 3 times the upper limit of normal) occur in jaundice owing to obstruction of the biliary system by pancreatic cancer, gallstones or secondary carcinoma and in primary biliary cirrhosis. More modest concentrations are found in hepatocellular disease due to viruses or alcohol. However, during a cholestatic phase of viral hepatitis, the alkaline phosphatase may reach very high levels.

Serum transaminases
Concentrations of transaminases in the plasma of more than 1000 iu are common in acute hepatitis from any cause. In

121

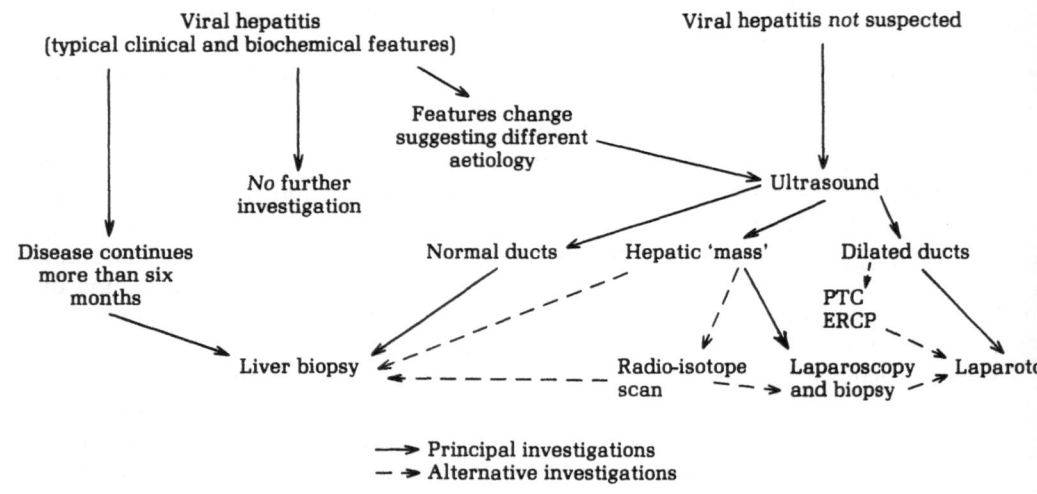

Diagnostic investigation of hepatocellular and cholestatic jaundice

Figure 11.1

biliary obstruction, levels tend to be considerably below this and may even be normal. Transaminase concentrations in cirrhosis and chronic hepatitis vary greatly from one patient to another. In chronic hepatitis levels are used to monitor activity of the disease and effectiveness of treatment.

Serum γ-glutamyl transpeptidase
    The concentration of γ-glutamyl transpeptidase tends to reflect that of alkaline phosphatase. When the level of this enzyme is raised and other enzyme concentrations are normal, alcoholic liver disease should be strongly suspected.

Plasma proteins
    Chronic hepatitis and cirrhosis are usually accompanied by low levels of albumin and raised concentrations of globulins. There is no diagnostically useful plasma protein pattern in acute hepatitis and obstructive jaundice.

Urine testing
    Bilirubinuria occurs in patients with jaundice due to hepatocellular disease and bile duct obstruction. It is not found in patients with haemolytic disease and unconjugated hyper-bilirubinaemias. Urobilinogen is absent from the urine in the presence of complete biliary tract obstruction.

Additional blood tests
    Hepatitis virus type B antigens (Australia antigen) and antibodies against this organism are present in the serum of patients with this disease. Patients with hepatitis due to type A virus have specific antibodies in the serum, but as yet this test is not generally available. The Paul–Bunnell test will be positive in the majority of patients with glandular fever.

Autoantibodies
The serum in cases of primary biliary cirrhosis almost invariably contains antimitochondrial antibodies. Smooth muscle antibodies are found in approximately 50% of patients with chronic active hepatitis.

Chest X-ray and GI endoscopy
If clinical evidence suggests secondary carcinoma, chest X-ray and endoscopic examination of the stomach may rapidly achieve a diagnosis.

Percutaneous liver biopsy
When the clinical and biochemical features indicate viral hepatitis further investigation is unnecessary. However, if jaundice persists or liver function tests fail to improve within six months of suggested viral hepatitis, liver biopsy should be obtained. This will enable distinction between chronic persistent hepatitis, which does not require specific treatment and chronic active hepatitis which does. Liver biopsy is also helpful in confirming suspected drug-induced jaundice. In the alcohol abuser severity of liver damage can be identified and a more accurate prognosis obtained. Micronodular cirrhosis can be diagnosed with accuracy by percutaneous needle biopsy because the abnormality tends to be diffuse. In contrast, macronodular cirrhosis may be missed by this technique as there are often large areas of liver where normal architecture is preserved. Histology of the liver will also separate jaundice due principally to hepatocellular disease from cholestatic conditions. In this latter group it is usually possible to distinguish primary biliary cirrhosis from other causes, but it is not always possible for the histopathologists to separate other causes of intrahepatic cholestasis from extrahepatic obstruction.

Laparoscopy
Laparoscopy can be performed following intravenous diazepam and local anaesthesia of the anterior abdominal wall. The hepatic surface can be inspected and biopsies of specific areas obtained under direct vision. It is therefore of particular value when carcinomatosis or macronodular cirrhosis is suspected.

Radio-isotope scanning
In cirrhosis, radioisotopes are taken up poorly by the liver, whereas the spleen has an increased avidity for the isotope. The technique is also useful for the detection of primary and secondary hepatic carcinomatous deposits.

Ultrasound screening
The increased sophistication of ultrasonic scanning has been a major advance in the management of jaundice. The principal benefit of ultrasound is its ability to detect dilated intra- and extrahepatic bile ducts. This enables patients with jaundice to be readily divided into those with an obstructive lesion of the large bile ducts, potentially amenable to surgery and those with other causes who do not require laparotomy. In

addition, ultrasonic scanning may show the cause of obstruction which is most commonly gallstone or carcinoma of the pancreas. When dilated ducts are not found this usually indicates an hepatic cause of jaundice and in these circumstances an experienced observer can usually distinguish cirrhosis from other pathologies.

Cholangio-
graphy
The routine oral cholecystogram and intravenous cholangiogram are of no use in the presence of hepatocellular and cholestatic jaundice because the radio-opaque medium is not secreted in sufficient concentration. There are two principal alternatives that can be used to demonstrate the biliary system.

Endoscopic retrograde cholangio-pancreatography (ERCP)

This involves the passage of a fine catheter through the biopsy channel of a flexible upper gastrointestinal endoscope into the ampulla of Vater. A radio-opaque medium is then injected into the biliary system. It will confirm or exclude dilatation and obstruction of the biliary ducts. This technique has two additional benefits. One is that the pancreatic ducts can also be examined which may reveal pancreatitis or carcinoma. The second advantage is the facility to remove stones from the common bile duct without the need for laparotomy.

Percutaneous transhepatic cholangiography (PTC)

This involves the passage of a very fine flexible needle through anaesthetized skin into the liver. When a bile duct is located, radio-opaque medium is injected which demonstrates either a dilated or normal biliary system. Patients in the former category are then referred for early surgery. The major advantage of this technique over ERCP is its relative simplicity, but it does not, of course, demonstrate the pancreatic ducts. In addition there is no facility for removal of stones but a modification of the method does allow a flexible drainage catheter to be percutaneously positioned in the liver so that jaundice can be temporarily relieved.

12 Miscellaneous gastrointestinal symptoms

Anorexia – The 'abnormal' tongue – Bad breath – Wind and gaseousness

Anorexia

It is important to distinguish between true loss of appetite and fear of eating because it causes pain or other symptoms. Restriction of food intake, due to precipitation of pain, is most commonly found in *peptic ulcer*. It also occurs in other conditions such as the *irritable bowel syndrome, mesenteric angina* and *pancreatitis*.

Malignant disease of almost any organ is accompanied by loss of appetite and weight loss, but is particularly marked in *carcinoma of the stomach*. Anorexia occurs, to a variable degree, in chronic debilitating conditions including *tuberculosis, Crohn's disease, uraemia* and *liver failure*, and may be the presenting symptom in *pernicious anaemia*.

Depression, particularly pathological grief, is often complicated by loss of desire to eat. Patients with *anorexia nervosa* do not usually complain of lost appetite. On the contrary, many will go to great lengths describing the foods they enjoy, but always fail to admit that only tiny amounts are taken and that carbohydrate is excluded (p. 35, 94).

In *pregnancy*, anorexia and nausea related to specific food items are probably far more common than the well recognized fads for bizarre foods.

125

The 'abnormal' tongue

Many patients become obsessed by what they consider to be an abnormality of their tongue. This may be either sensation or appearance. *Burning* is the commonest complaint but in only one of five patients can a cause for the symptom be found. Deficiencies of folic acid and the vitamin B complex, including B_{12}, give rise to a sore, red and depapillated tongue. In others there may be dental disorders, excessive smoking or recent treatment with antibiotics, all of which should be obvious from the history or examination. The great majority have no identifiable abnormality. In such patients there is usually a long history and multiple attendances to medical and dental clinics. Reassurance, particularly about the absence of cancer, is all that can be offered. The commonest complaint about appearance of the tongue is *coating. A white or yellow coat on the tongue is a physiological phenomenon.* It consists of food debris, desquamated epithelium and bacteria. It is most obvious in the morning and is encouraged by mouth breathing, fasting and smoking. A combination of the first two causes is the likely explanation for the coated tongue seen in pyrexial diseases. *Black coating* of the tongue is thought to be due to bacterial or fungal proliferation and is particularly common after antibiotic therapy. It is harmless, resolves spontaneously and, like physiological coating, requires no specific treatment.

Fissuring and discovery of the *large circumvalate papillae* at the back of the tongue often alarm patients. Strong reassurance solves the problem in the great majority of cases. *Aphthous ulcers* may affect the tongue as well as the buccal mucosa. The aetiology is unknown.

General debility, emotional stress and local irritation appear to be aetiological factors, but association with other diseases is non-specific. Healing is spontaneous and topical steroids, carbenoxylone and disodium cromoglycate have never been shown conclusively to enhance resolution.

In a few patients complaining of symptoms involving the tongue, examination will reveal disease requiring further investigation and more definitive treatment. These include *carcinomatous ulcers, leukoplakia* and *macroglossia* due to *amyloidosis* or *myxoedema*.

Bad breath

A distinction should be made between bad breath that can be smelt by others and that of which only the patient is aware. The latter is often combined with a 'bad taste' in the mouth and is frequently part of an obsessional neurosis. Thorough examination, reassurance and encouragement to continue with normal, but not excessive, oral toilet will satisfy many patients. Only in occasional cases will referral to a psychiatrist be either necessary or helpful.

Halitosis, on first waking, should be regarded as normal and is likely to be most severe in mouth breathers and smokers. Cleaning the teeth and eating breakfast usually solve the problem. Bad breath at other times of the day is commonly due to dental and gingival disease, combined with poor oral hygiene. Odours on the breath resulting from specific food items, such as garlic and onions, are obvious and the cure is self-evident. Fats and meat proteins are other possible sources of odoriferous, volatile metabolic products excreted in the breath. If the symptom is particularly troublesome a reduction in dietary animal products is worth trying.

Neoplastic or chronic sepsis of the nasopharynx and lungs may give rise to an unpleasant odour but this is insignificant compared with other symptoms. Similarly, although helpful in making a clinical diagnosis, the feotors of ketosis, uraemia and hepatic failure are rarely remarked upon by the patient.

Bad breath is not an indication of bowel disease per se *or the result of constipation.*

Wind and gaseousness

'Excessive gas' in the alimentary tract is a common complaint. The most frequent symptoms are belching, passing 'excessive' flatus, a feeling of abdominal distension with inability to pass flatus, colicky pain and borborygmi.

Oxygen, nitrogen, hydrogen, carbon dioxide and methane contribute 99% of the gas in the alimentary tract. *Swallowed air* is the major source of oxygen and nitrogen. Hydrogen and methane are produced by bacteria. The majority of carbon dioxide is also endogenous, arising from both bacterial fermentation and acidification of bicarbonate-containing secretions. Very small quantities of highly odoriferous gases produced by colonic bacteria make up the remaining 1%.

The mechanism of excess gas production in many conditions can be explained. In *small bowel diverticulosis* the cause is bacterial proliferation, whereas *small intestinal malabsorption* and maldigestion due to *pancreatic disease* result in an increased substrate for colonic bacteria. Successful management depends upon treatment of the underlying condition. By contrast, in the great majority of patients with symptoms of gaseousness no underlying pathology is evident. Except in pyloric stenosis, no appreciable amounts of gas are produced by bacteria in the stomach. Thus, *patients with belching as their main complaint almost invariably practice aerophagy.* This is frequently a feature of *anxiety.* It is also seen in patients with oesophagitis who develop the habit of swallowing saliva to neutralize irritant gastric acid refluxed into the distal oesophagus. Irritant mouth lesions, *chewing gum* or *eating and drinking too quickly* may also encourage air to be taken into the stomach. Although most of this excess air is belched out, some undoubtedly passes distally and contributes to the other symptoms of gaseousness. These include the *feeling of abdominal distension and pain* which arise mainly from the small intestine or colon. Experimental evidence suggests that *in most patients with these symptoms there is no excess of gastrointestinal gas.* The major problem is an inability to accommodate normal volumes without pain being produced. These patients also often have a slow transit time through the gut and gas appears to collect in the splenic and hepatic flexures. Gaseousness is a common component of the irritable bowel syndrome.

Curing belching depends upon treatment of underlying anxiety and correction of the other factors which encourage aerophagy. These should also be looked for in patients complaining of abdominal distension, pain and borborygmi. Although excess production of gas does not appear to be the basic pathogenic mechanism in such patients, measures that reduce flatus formation often help. It hardly needs to be mentioned that certain vegetables, such as cabbage and beans, promote intestinal gas production. Less well appreciated is that apple juice, grape juice, raisins and bananas have a similar effect. Dietary manipulation is, therefore, worthy of trial. Attempts to alleviate symptoms by changing intestinal bacterial flora with antibiotics has not met with any consistent success. Similarly, claims that charcoal, kaolin, dimethicone and chlorophyll are beneficial have not been substantiated.

⅓ Gastrointestinal endoscopy

The flexible fibrescope has now made it possible to examine the gastrointestinal tract from the oesophagus to the anus. Initially, the main use for the fibrescope was diagnostic, but during the past few years a growing range of therapeutic procedures has been developed. Diagnosis is made by the clear visualization of lesions combined with tissue biopsy and brush cytology. The therapeutic procedures include insertion of oesophageal tubes, injection of oesophageal varices, removal of foreign bodies, clipping and photocoagulation of gastric bleeding points, papillotomy for retained stones and colonic and gastric polypectomy.

Equipment

Although the invention of a flexible fibre optic image bundle was made in Britain, at the present time only Japanese and American endoscopes are available. Production costs now make it unlikely that there will ever be a British fibrescope. There is a vast array of instruments to choose from; however, the standard endoscope has many common features. The lengths vary from 1 to 2 metres with an outside diameter of 10–13 mm. The proximal control mechanism allows manipulation of the very flexible distal tip up to 180° in all directions. The shaft of the instrument contains one or more light bundles for the transmission of light from a separate source and a coherent viewing fibre bundle for transmission of the image. The proximal control mechanism allows the insufflation of air and the suction of air and fluids. The tip of the instrument is cleaned by a small jet of water.

UPPER GASTROINTESTINAL ENDOSCOPY

Advice to patients undergoing upper GI endoscopy

Apprehension is common to most patients undergoing endoscopy. Strong reassurance will allay most of the anxieties. Patients are advised to fast overnight or for 6–8 hours prior to endoscopy. Diazepam (Valium) 10–30 mg intravenously is used for sedation. Atropine may be of help to dry local secretions. Local anaesthetic pharyngeal spray may also be used. Drugs such as glucagon or an anti-cholinergic may be necessary for complete examination of the duodenum. As the majority of endoscopies are done as outpatient procedures, it is advisable to keep the medication to a minimum. Patients are allowed to recover for 1 or 2 hours on a bed or a trolley. They should be accompanied home by a friend or relative and not allowed to drive a car.

Failures and complications

A small proportion of patients – approximately 1% – require a general anaesthetic. Such patients include the heavy drinker and occasionally a very anxious patient. At all other times gentleness and care should be exercised both for the patient and the instruments. Serious complications fortunately are rare; they include perforation of the oesophagus and aspiration pneumonitis.

Indications

The majority of endoscopies are a direct result of a radiological finding. However, many endoscopists will proceed without resorting to X-rays. At the present time, radiology and endoscopy provide a complementary diagnostic service.

Contraindications

These are few and include thoracic aortic aneurysm, a positive Australia antigen and tuberculosis.

Oesophagus

Indications are:

(1) Dysphagia
(2) Hiatus hernia and heartburn
(3) Radiological lesions
(4) Upper gastrointestinal bleeding.

Gastrointestinal endoscopy

Hiatus hernia and oesophagitis

Radiography can demonstrate hiatus hernia and reflux, but it is of little value in demonstrating oesophagitis. Endoscopy and biopsy will confirm the extent and the severity of the oesophagitis. Symptomatically, however, there is no direct relationship between the degree of oesophagitis and the severity of symptoms. Symptomatic patients with no endoscopic or biopsy evidence of oesophagitis should be further investigated for other causative lesions such as gallbladder disease or coronary artery disease.

Dysphagia

All patients with dysphagia should have an endoscopy. If there is any suggestion of achalasia or pharyngeal pouch in the history, it is important that the patient should have a barium meal before endoscopy. In the majority of cases the diagnosis rests between (1) a malignant stricture or a benign stricture secondary to a hiatus hernia and (2) achalasia. The diagnosis of achalasia can be made by radiological and manometric examination but endoscopy is able to exclude a benign or malignant stricture. Endoscopy and biopsy allow an accurate diagnosis to be made and the appropriate treatment to be planned.

Dilatation of oesophageal stricture

Benign and malignant strictures may be dilated with an Eder Peustow dilator. This technique using a flexible gastroscope is much safer than the older method with a rigid oesophagoscope. A fine guide wire is passed down the biopsy channel of the gastroscope through the stricture. The gastroscope is withdrawn leaving the guide wire in situ. A series of graduated bougies are passed over the guide wire through the stricture. Benign oesophageal strictures, particularly in the elderly patient, may be managed successfully for many years. Malignant strictures may require dilatation prior to the insertion of oesophageal tube.

Insertion of oesophageal tubes

Malignant or intractable fibrous strictures may be treated by inserting an oesophageal tube endoscopically through the

131

strictures. Elderly inoperable or poor-risk patients do badly from more conventional methods of inserting oesophageal tube, i.e. laparotomy and gastrostomy. Although the prognosis in patients with malignant strictures is poor, their final months can be made more comfortable by the per oral insertion of an oesophageal tube. A small group of patients may respond to radiotherapy with the oesophageal tube *in situ*.

Fibre optic injection of oesophageal varices

Oesophageal varices respond poorly to shunting procedures both in the bleeding and elective patient. Recent studies have emphasized the value of sclerotherapy in patients who have bled from oesophageal varices. The original method described used a rigid oesophagoscope and a long rigid injection needle. More recently the fibrescope has been used in conjunction with an outer sheath. A small window in the distal end of the sheath isolates each varix separately. The sclerosant is injected directly into each varix by a long flexible needle introduced down the biopsy channel of the gastroscope.

Stomach

Indications are:

(1) Barium meal negative dyspepsia
(2) Gastric ulcer
(3) Gastrointestinal bleeding
(4) Postgastrectomy problems.

Symptomatic patients who have a negative barium meal and cholecystogram often present difficult problems in management. Over 50% of the patients will have a positive endoscopic lesion; these lesions include gastritis, duodenitis, small peptic ulcers, oesophagitis and early carcinoma. Negative endoscopy often helps to reassure both the patient and the doctor.

Gastric ulcer

All patients with gastric ulcers should have an endoscopy. Unfortunately, radiology is not able to determine accurately whether an ulcer is benign or malignant. A small proportion of radiologically benign ulcers will on biopsy be malignant (3–10%). It is advisable that all patients with gastric ulcers should have gastroscopy done on several occasions. This allows healing to be checked and also the occasional missed malignant ulcer to be spotted.

Gastric carcinoma

Endoscopy is helpful in this group of patients in that it gives accurate histological confirmation prior to surgery. The extent of the proximal spread may also influence operability.

Duodenum

Modern oesophago-gastro-duodenoscopy includes accurate visualization of the duodenum. Occasionally pyloric stenosis makes this impossible.

Indications are:

(1) Barium meal negative dyspepsia
(2) Equivocal radiology
(3) Duodenitis
(4) Gastrointestinal bleeding
(5) Perspective studies of duodenal ulcer healing
(6) Prior to surgery.

Patients with typical symptoms of duodenal ulceration and X-ray confirmation of the ulcer should be treated medically without resorting to endoscopy. Repeated follow-up endoscopy is only useful in drug trials.

Gastrointestinal bleeding

All patients with upper gastrointestinal bleeding should have an endoscopy, unless there is a strong medical contraindication. Diagnostic accuracy exceeds 90% if performed within 24 h. The common causes include bleeding duodenal ulcers, gastric ulcers, acute erosions, oesophageal varices, Mallory–Weiss syndrome and carcinoma. Endoscopic methods of arresting gastrointestinal bleeding have been, and are being, evaluated. They include the application of metal clips, electro-coagulation and laser photocoagulation.

Achalasia

Pneumatic dilatation of the distal oesophagus in achalasia has been performed for many years, but over the past 10 years has gained in popularity. The dilatation is performed with the patient sitting in the upright position. An inflatable balloon is passed to the lower end of the oesophagus and gradually inflated. Several dilatations are usually required and the success of the treatment is determined by manometric and X-ray examinations. The long term results appear to be comparable to those obtained by the Heller's operation. Those who support pneumatic dilatation as the treatment of choice for achalasia feel that surgery is indicated (1) after several unsuccessful attempts at pneumatic dilatation, (2) when oesophageal carcinoma cannot be excluded and (3) in children and psychiatric patients who are unable to co-operate.

Therapeutic endoscopy

Therapeutic endoscopy – intubation of malignant oesophago-gastric strictures – this is basically a palliative procedure to relieve distressing dysphagia. The average survival time after oesophageal intubation is 3 months. Endoscopic intubation is a new procedure and is rapidly gaining in popularity over the conventional operative intubation. The advantages of endoscopic intubation over operative intubation are the lower immediate mortality and the avoidance of wound infection. One main disadvantage is tube displacement. The oesophageal tube is stitched securely to the stomach wall in the operative method. This helps prevent migration of the tube either back into the oesophagus or down into the stomach. Recent new designs in oesophageal tubes have a flange at the lower end which helps prevent tube displacement back into the oesophagus.

Method of intubation

The procedure is carried out under general or local anaesthesia. A flexible guide wire is placed down the biopsy channel of the gastroscope through the malignant stricture. The stricture is dilated with Eder Peustow dilators until a large enough channel is obtained through the oesophageal tube. With the guide wire still in place, a plastic prosthesis is introduced into the lower end of the oesophagus and lodged firmly within the stricture. A variety of introducers are available for inserting the oesophageal tube.

Advice to patients

Patients are advised to eat soft or well-masticated food. It is worth advising the patient that the internal diameter of the tube is about the same size as an adult index finger. Drinks such as soda water and lemonade must be taken after each meal to wash out any remaining food debris within the tube. Acid reflux may become a troublesome problem and patients are advised to sleep with two or three pillows. Symptoms of oesophagitis respond in the majority of patients to a combination of alkali and an H_2 antagonist such as cimetidine. In a small group of patients this remains a resistant troublesome problem.

Oesophageal intubation and radiotherapy

The overall prognosis in squamous cell carcinoma of the oeso-phagus is poor. However, dysphagia caused by a malignant stricture of the lower third of the oesophagus will often respond to radiotherapy. These tumours may be intubated prior to radio-therapy and a full course of radiotherapy given with the tube *in situ*. It may then be possible to remove the tube following completion of treatment.

COLONOSCOPY

Modern fibre optic colonoscopy has enabled the colon to be fully examined from the anus to the caecum. It is without doubt the most accurate way of making a diagnosis of a colonic lesion. Colonoscopy is invariably preceded by a good double-contrast barium enema and rigid sigmoidoscopy.

Patient preparation

Good colonoscopy can only be performed with an adequately cleaned colon. All patients require some type of bowel prepar-ation. This entails a combination of a fluid diet, purgation and enemata. Whether or not it is done as an in-patient or out-patient depends very much on the experience of the colon-oscopist.

Sedation

The majority of colonoscopies are performed with intravenous Valium 5–20 mg as sedation, and pethidine 50–100 mg intra-venously or Fortral 30 mg intravenously for analgesia. It is not necessary for a patient to be given a general anaesthetic.

Indications for colonoscopy

(1) Evaluation of barium enema abnormalities. Mucosal abnormalities, filling defects and strictures of the colon will often require a colonoscopy to determine their exact cause. This is particularly true in the sigmoid colon and caecum. Colonoscopy is often helpful in differentiating malignant from inflammatory strictures due to diverticular disease and confirming the absence or presence of a possible polyp.

(2) Evaluation of unexplained rectal bleeding. Patients who have a negative barium enema and sigmoidoscopy may benefit from a colonoscopy. The patients will have presented with obvious blood in the stool, or positive occult blood or occasionally an unexplained anaemia. On colonoscopy a significant number will be found to have a colonic polyp, carcinoma, inflammatory bowel disease, or angio-dysplasia. The source of massive rectal bleeding is difficult to evaluate at the time of the bleed. However, as colonic bleeding tends to be intermittent, it may be possible to determine the cause after the the bleeding has stopped. The common causes are diverticular disease, colonic polyps, carcinoma and angiodysplasia.

Massive rectal bleeding

(3) Inflammatory bowel disease. Most patients with inflammatory bowel disease will not require a colonoscopy. It may, however, be useful in differentiating Crohn's disease from ulcerative colitis. Most barium enemata examinations underestimate the extent of ulcerative colitis and Crohn's disease. Colonoscopy may be helpful in evaluating the true extent of the disease.

(4) Follow-up of colonic polyps. Patients who have had a previous polypectomy are advised to have a good barium enema or colonoscopy every two/three years. The incidence of recurrent polyps is significantly higher in this group than the normal population.

Therapeutic colonoscopy

(1) Colonoscopic polypectomy. This procedure has now dramatically changed the management of colonic polyps. Until quite recently these have been treated by laparotomy with colonic resection or colotomy. The technique itself is quite simple, although considerable experience is required in its application. The polyp is gripped by an electrode snare

which is passed through the biopsy channel of the colon-oscope. The polyp is removed by tightening the snare and electrocoagulating the base of the polyp. Piecemeal removal may be required for larger polyps. This technique has markedly reduced the cost, morbidity and mortality in the management of colonic polyps.

(2) Management of colonic bleeding. The techniques available for stopping colonic bleeding are electrocoagulation or photocoagulation. Both these techniques have found limited applications at the present time. Also photocoagulation using a laser beam is for most colonoscopists prohibitively expensive.

Colonoscopy in general practice

Colonoscopy is now freely available in most hospitals. Family doctors should have no hesitation in referring patients for colonoscopy, if they think it is clinically indicated and if a high quality double contrast barium enema has not produced a diagnosis.

Part 2
Common diseases

14 Peptic ulcer

Aetiological factors – Clinical features – Diagnosis – Management

The commonest sites of peptic ulceration are the duodenum and stomach. Ulcers occur less frequently in the oesophagus as a complication of gastro-oesophageal reflux and at the anastomosis of stomach and intestinal mucosa following gastric surgery. Peptic ulcer is a worldwide disease. In the United Kingdom, duodenal ulcer has an annual incidence of more than two per 1000 in men and 0.62 per 1000 in women. Gastric ulcer is less common, the figures being 0.53 per 1000 for men and 0.31 per 1000 in women. It has been estimated that at some time in their life one in five men and one in ten women develop a peptic ulcer. Although duodenal and gastric ulcer are both very common diseases it seems likely that the incidence of both has decreased during the past 25 years. The reasons are not clear. Both gastric and duodenal ulcers are more common in UK social classes 4 and 5 than in those with professional and managerial occupations.

Pathogenesis   Ulceration occurs when the gastroduodenal mucosa breaks down under the erosive effect of gastric acid and pepsin. Although acid production is necessary for the production of *gastric ulceration*, excessive amounts are not found. It seems likely that bile refluxed from the duodenum is an equally important factor. Gastric stasis may also play a role. A diffuse gastritis is almost invariable in patients with gastric ulcer but it is not known why only small areas actually ulcerate. Relative ischaemia due to the vascular architecture of the stomach may

141

be the underlying mechanism for this, which might explain why the lesser curve is so commonly affected.

Following stimulation with pentagastrin, excessive gastric acid production is found in 30–40% of patients with *duodenal ulcer*. Probably of more importance is that the majority of duodenal ulcer patients secrete an inappropriately high quantity of acid between meals and at night. This implies that the normal control mechanisms for gastric acid synthesis are defective. In this context, there is evidence that in duodenal ulcer there may be an inappropriate production of the stimulatory hormone gastrin or increased sensitivity of parietal cells to its action.

It is possible that pepsin may also damage the upper gastrointestinal mucosa and recent work has shown an increased secretion of this enzyme during the active phase of duodenal ulceration. Another possible factor in duodenal ulcer is defective neutralization of gastric acid. This could result from inadequate mixing of acid with food due to rapid emptying of the stomach, which is a feature found in many duodenal ulcer patients. An alternative mechanism is failure of the pancreas to produce sufficient bicarbonate to neutralize gastric acid, a phenomenon often found in duodenal ulcer.

Compared with the study of erosive factors there has been relatively little investigation of mucus or the mucosal epithelium in peptic ulcer. As yet there is no conclusive evidence that either is abnormal. Urogastrone, a substance produced by mammalian salivary glands, inhibits gastric secretion. It has been suggested that deficiency of this substance could predispose to peptic ulceration.

Aetiological factors

Genetic factors
: Blood group O or the failure to produce blood group substances in mucous secretions is associated with a higher risk of both duodenal and gastric ulcer. That genetic components have a role is also supported by the higher incidence of duodenal ulceration in monozygotic twins compared to dizygotic twins.

Diet
: No dietary item has been conclusively identified as a cause of ulcer. It has been suggested that a 'refined' diet predisposes to the disease, but evidence is lacking. A diet requiring mastication may be protective because it stimulates saliva which, in turn, neutralizes gastric acid and delays gastric emptying.

Alcohol
: There is no evidence that alcohol in moderation causes either gastric or duodenal ulcers.

142

Peptic ulcer

Coffee

There is evidence that duodenal ulcer is related to excessive drinking of coffee and specific advice to avoid this should be given.

Smoking

Smokers have peptic ulcers more commonly than non-smokers. Healing, especially of gastric ulcer, is delayed by continuing to smoke.

Drugs

Aspirin has been implicated as a cause of gastric ulcer. Women who have taken continuous excessive quantities seem to be particularly at risk. Although anti-inflammatory drugs, such as phenylbutazone and corticosteroids, can induce acute ulcers in experimental animals, there is no definite evidence that they are a major cause of chronic ulceration in man.

Psychological factors

Emotion has a profound influence on alimentary tract function including gastric secretion and motility, but there is little to support the concept of an 'ulcer personality'. Nevertheless, it is possible that 'stress' may be an exacerbating factor in an individual prone to peptic ulcer.

Clinical features

Pain

Pain in the epigastrium is the characteristic symptom of peptic ulcer. It may be experienced less often in the hypochondria or around the umbilicus. Only in rare cases does it give rise to lower abdominal pain. Radiation to the back and chest is common. The pain is most frequently described as gnawing, knife-like, a deep ache, tearing or severe hunger. *The intensity of pain bears no relationship to the size of an ulcer and increased severity does not indicate incipient perforation or haemorrhage.* Pain is unrelated to meals in 50% of patients with duodenal ulcer. In the remainder, food may either precipitate or relieve symptoms. Antacids give more consistent relief but are completely effective in only 40%. *Pain which wakes the patient from sleep in the early hours of the morning is present in 70% of duodenal ulcer cases and in 30% of those with gastric ulcer.* Attacks last from 1 to 4 weeks and are followed by remission of several weeks or months.

Vomiting and reflux

Vomiting may occur during severe bouts of pain. It may sometimes be induced because it affords relief. *Vomiting does not necessarily indicate pyloric obstruction.* Reflux of gastric contents into the oesophagus occurs commonly in duodenal ulcer and may cause heartburn or the appearance of acid or bile in the mouth.

Weight loss

During exacerbations mild weight loss is frequently observed, but the weight is rapidly regained when in remission.

143

This contrasts with the progressive and profound loss of weight seen with gastric carcinoma.

Examination   In uncomplicated cases the only physical sign is tenderness in the epigastrium.

In an individual patient duodenal ulcer cannot definitely be distinguished from ulceration of the stomach on clinical evidence alone.

Diagnosis

Endoscopy and radiology   *Barium meal* is still the most commonly requested investigation in those suspected of peptic ulcer. Nevertheless, it must be remembered that posterior wall gastric ulcers and those in the second part of the duodenum are easily missed. Scarring of the duodenal cap, from previous ulceration, also makes radiological diagnosis of active ulceration more difficult. *Endoscopy* is less likely to miss such lesions and in most established centres more than 90% of all peptic ulcers will be identified. *If the barium meal shows a duodenal ulcer, endoscopy is not necessary.* Although an experienced radiologist can usually distinguish gastric ulcer from cancer, *it is now common practice to use endoscopy and biopsy in all patients with gastric lesions.*

Gastric secretion tests   Gastric secretion studies are of no major diagnostic value and are no longer used in routine investigation.

Management

The generally accepted aims of treatment are relief of symptoms, to heal the ulcer and if possible prevent relapse. Many varying forms of therapy have been carefully studied during the past 30 years.

Diet   *So-called 'gastric diets' have not been shown to heal peptic ulcers.* Nevertheless, the patient often adopts a regime of small regular meals because of the symptomatic relief that it achieves. Many also avoid certain substances such as fats and alcohol because they exacerbate their symptoms. Milk frequently provides effective temporary relief from pain.

Bed rest   Rest in bed relieves the symptoms of both gastric and duodenal ulcers. However, enhancement of healing has only been demonstrated in gastric ulcer. Since the advent of effective drug therapy it is now rarely necessary.

Smoking   As yet there is no conclusive proof that smoking directly increases the risk of developing peptic ulcer. In contrast, ceasing to smoke accelerates gastric ulcer healing, although in duodenal ulcer it has a less obvious effect.

Histamine H₂ antagonists

At present two drugs, cimetidine (Tagamet) and ranitidine (Zantac are available in the histamine H_2 antagonist group. They work by blocking the H_2 receptors on gastric parietal cells through which histamine exerts its secretory effect. They are now established as the drugs of first choice in ulcer treatment. Many trials have confirmed that a 4–6 week course accelerates healing of both gastric and duodenal ulcer. There appears to be no marked difference in their healing capacity compared with carbenoxolone or De-Nol (bismuth salts, see below) but they more rapidly control symptoms. Unwanted effects are rare. A few patients on cimetidine have developed diarrhoea, skin rash or muscle pain. Confusion in elderly patients has also been reported. A very small number of patients on long term treatment have noticed gynaecomastia, loss of libido and impotence. These effects are reversed on withdrawal of the drug. As yet there have been no consistent reports of serious side effects in patients on ranitidine.

Antacids

For many years antacids have been the mainstay of ulcer treatment. Until very recently no healing effect had been shown and their efficacy was based upon symptom relief. When antacids are used for this purpose, the patient should take regular doses between meals and before retiring at night. He should also be encouraged to take as many additional doses as necessary to keep himself free of pain. Recent studies have shown that in very large doses a combination of magnesium and aluminium hydroxides accelerates duodenal ulcer healing. The amounts of antacid involved and the looseness of stool caused by the regime make it unacceptable for general use. *Sodium bicarbonate* should never be used on a long term basis because it can cause metabolic alkalosis. *Aluminium salts* often constipate and *magnesium compounds* cause diarrhoea. Preparations containing a combination of these substances are therefore advisable. *Calcium salts*, although they rapidly neutralize hydrochloric acid, should be avoided because calcium stimulates gastrin secretion and leads to a rebound hypersecretion of acid.

Anticholinergic drugs

Drugs in the anticholinergic group when given intravenously or in large oral doses significantly reduce gastric secretion. However, at these levels side-effects such as blurred vision, dry mouth and drowsiness are inevitable. The development of H_2 histamine antagonists has made these drugs virtually obsolete in the treatment of peptic ulcer.

Carben-oxolone

Carbenoxolone is derived from glycyrrhizinic acid which occurs naturally in liquorice. It has no signficant antisecretory action and is effective because it 'strengthens' the gastro-duodenal mucosa. It does so by increasing mucus production and prolonging mucosal cell life. Both gastric and duodenal ulcer healing is accelerated. The preparation used in gastric ulcer in Biogastrone and in duodenal ulcer is Duogastrone. The latter is in a capsule form which is said to deliver the compound in high concentration to the duodenal mucosa. A 4–6 week course is sufficient in the majority of patients. Fluid and sodium retention, hypertension and hypokalaemia are major unwanted effects. Because of this, many practitioners now prescribe potassium supplements and a thiazide diuretic in conjunction with carbenoxolone. If these additional preparations are not given, the patient's blood pressure and cardiovascular status should be reviewed weekly. The risk is greatest in the elderly and, with the advent of cimetidine, their use in this age group is no longer advised.

Deglycyr-rhizinated liquorice

Both Caved-(S) and Ulcedal appear to have some ulcer healing effect but are less potent than carbenoxolone. They do not cause fluid retention and electrolyte disturbance and can, therefore, be used freely in the elderly. When they are used in high dosage, diarrhoea may be a problem.

Bismuth salts

Tripotassium dicitrato bismuthate in a colloidal alkalinated solution (De-Nol) promotes the healing of peptic ulcers. Treatment is usually required for 4–6 weeks. The method of action is not clear but is thought to include precipitation of bismuth with the proteinatious exudate of the ulcer which forms a protective film, stimulation of mucus and an antipepsin activity. It has no significant side-effects but many patients find the ammoniacal smell difficult to tolerate.

Other compounds

A number of alternative compounds are currently being studied.

Antipepsins

In contrast to hydrochloric acid, the ulcerogenic properties of pepsin have not been extensively investigated, but it is likely that this enzyme does have a role in the production of peptic ulcer. A number of 'antipepsins' have been developed but, as yet, there is no conclusive evidence of their effectiveness in healing ulcers.

Prosta-glandins

Prostaglandins are a group of naturally occurring cyclic fatty acids which have a very wide range of activity. One group inhibits gastric secretion. A synthetic analogue has been shown to heal duodenal and gastric ulcers but it is not yet freely available.

146

Peptic ulcer

Proglumide

Proglumide inhibits gastric secretion probably by competitive inhibition of gastrin. It accelerates the healing of duodenal ulcer but it has not been promoted in the United Kingdom.

Prevention of relapse

There is no doubt that cimetidine, ranitidine, carbenoxylone and De-Nol promote the healing of peptic ulcer. It is doubtful whether H_2 antagonists change the natural history of ulcer disease and relapse frequently occurs within a few weeks of stopping treatment. This has led to the search for a prophylactic regime. In this context, cimetidine 200 mg twice daily or 400 mg at night has proved very successful. In patients with long spontaneous symptomatic remissions, however, prophylactic therapy is probably not justified. Instead, each relapse should be treated with a 4–6 week course of the drug. Long term prophylactic therapy should be reserved for those patients who are experiencing severe and frequent relapses. Failure to achieve symptomatic relief with full doses of cimetidine, or frequent relapse whilst on long term, low dose cimetidine, is a strong indication to consider surgery.

Recent studies suggest that ulcers healed with the aid of De-Nol and perhaps high dose antacids remain in remission longer than those healed with the assistance of cimetidine. Confirmation of these findings is awaited.

Points to stress

Characteristics of pain due to peptic ulcer

- Individual attacks usually last only a few hours
- Tend to occur daily for several days
- Frequently nocturnal
- Relieved by antacids
- Freedom from severe symptoms for several weeks or months.

Persisting epigastric pain, plus anorexia and weight loss indicates gastric cancer

OPERATIONS FOR PEPTIC ULCERATION

Duodenal ulcer

The surgical procedures currently used are:—

Truncal or selective vagotomy with pyloroplasty, gastrojejunostomy or antrectomy.

147

Subtotal gastrectomy of the Bilroth II type and highly selective vagotomy.

It is beyond the scope of this book to discuss the merits of each operation. However, some general comments can be made.

There has been an increasing trend towards surgical conservatism. The ideal operation should have no mortality, minimal morbidity and no recurrent ulceration. The morbidity associated with gastric operations includes dumping, diarrhoea, biliary reflux, and long term nutritional problems. Partial gastrectomy, vagotomy and antrectomy have a very low incidence of recurrent ulceration but significant morbidity and mortality.

Vagotomy and pyloroplasty or gastro-jejunostomy have a low morbidity and mortality but a significant incidence of recurrent ulceration. These two operations are the most commonly performed procedures for uncomplicated duodenal ulceration.

The recently introduced highly selective vagotomy holds most hope for the future. The morbidity and mortality associated with the operation are very low. The short term recurrent ulceration rate appears encouragingly low. Several large clinical trials are currently evaluating this operation.

Gastric ulcer

The standard operation for an uncomplicated gastric ulcer is a Bilroth I gastrectomy. However, there is increasing evidence that the lesser procedure of highly selective vagotomy may be adequate in most patients.

15 Some diseases that cause malabsorption

<hr>

Coeliac disease – Malabsorption after gastric surgery – Crohn's disease – Malabsorption after small bowel resection – Small intestinal lymphoma – Chronic small bowel ischaemia – Bacterial colonization of small intestine – Post-infective malabsorption – Giardiasis – Tropical sprue – Whipple's disease – Pancreatic insufficiency

The clinical features and investigation of patients with malabsorption have been described (p. 84). The purpose of this chapter is to discuss more fully the aetiology, pathogenesis and specific management of some diseases that cause the malabsorption syndrome.

Coeliac disease

Coeliac disease, which is also called 'coeliac sprue' and 'gluten sensitive enteropathy', is caused by the toxic effect of gluten on the small intestinal mucosa. The mechanism by which gluten induces damage is not known. Two main theories have been proposed. One is that the small intestinal mucosa in coeliac disease is deficient in an enzyme which normally digests gluten and renders it 'non-toxic'. The second is that patients with coeliac disease mount an immunological response against gluten which damages the mucosa. This theory is supported by the fact that certain HLA tissue-type antigens which are associated with immunological disorders are also very commonly

149

found in coeliac disease. Furthermore, immunological dysfunction and autoimmune diseases occur with increased prevalence in coeliac disease.

In Britain approximately one in 2000 of the population is thought to have the disorder, but in the west of Ireland the figure may be as high as one in 400. There is undoubtedly an increased familial incidence, but the genetic mode of inheritance is not clear.

Diagnosis can be made only by small bowel biopsy. The dissecting microscope shows the absence of normal finger and leaf shaped villi. Varying degrees of villous atrophy, shortening of the normally columnar enterocytes and a heavy inflammatory infiltrate of the epithelium and lamina propria are seen on histology. It has recently become common practice to ensure that the mucosa has returned towards normal by obtaining a second biopsy after several months' therapy.

Treatment is by exclusion of gluten from the diet. This involves avoidance of products made with wheat, barley and rye flour. Whether oats are toxic remains unclear, but maize flour is certainly safe. Once established, the diet is easily managed, unless meals are frequently taken in restaurants. A large variety of gluten-free foods are now on the market, many of which are obtainable in the UK on NHS prescription. Information about these can be obtained from The Coeliac Society.

Many patients require no encouragement to remain on their diet, because it makes them feel better or a relapse is experienced if they fail to do so. Children are very rarely unresponsive to the diet, but many adults appear to take much longer before symptoms resolve and normal nutrition is achieved. The commonest reason for failure to respond is non-compliance but a few patients, even after prolonged inpatient supervision of dietary treatment, remain unresponsive. If significant symptoms persist in this group, the use of steroids is justified; this frequently leads to nutritional and histological improvement. If malabsorption continues, small bowel lymphoma or additional pancreatic impairment must be considered. Initially, it is often necessary to correct nutritional deficiencies, especially iron and folate, but as small intestinal function improves these supplements should not be required. Some patients refuse to remain on a strict gluten free regime and they may need long term iron and folate supplements to prevent anaemia. Coeliac disease in adult life is associated with an increased incidence of small intestinal lymphoma and carcinoma. Cancer of the oesophagus is also more common in this disease than in the general population. Another rarer complication is ulceration of the small bowel. There is no conclusive evidence that the incidence of either malignancy or ulceration is reduced by a gluten-free diet.

Dermatitis herpetiformis

A small intestinal lesion identical to that of coeliac disease is found in the great majority of patients with *dermatitis herpetiformis*. This skin condition is characterized by an irritant vesicular rash. In contrast to coeliac disease, gut symptoms and clinical nutritional disturbance are relatively rare. Nevertheless, if the patient is willing, a gluten-free diet should be tried because both the gut and skin lesions are responsive to this treatment. The alternative therapy for the rash is dapsone, but this has no effect upon the bowel abnormality.

Malabsorption after gastric surgery

The mechanisms leading to malabsorption after gastric surgery have been discussed (p. 83). Iron deficiency anaemia is the commonest nutritional disturbance following gastrectomy. It is mainly due to malabsorption, but in many patients bleeding from gastritis or recurrent ulceration contribute. Reduction of intrinsic factor synthesis following gastric resection impairs vitamin B_{12} absorption. Mild degrees of steatorrhoea are common but postgastrectomy diarrhoea is only rarely due to this mechanism. However, patients with a blind loop syndrome, due to a previous Polya gastrectomy, may have symptomatic steatorrhoea.

All patients after gastric surgery should have an annual haemoglobin estimation. Any tendency to anaemia should be further investigated and serum levels of iron and vitamin B_{12} measured. Iron deficiency can usually be corrected by oral preparations and only rarely requires parenteral replacement. In contrast, vitamin B_{12} must always be administered by the intramuscular route. Following total gastrectomy these deficiencies are inevitable and should be prevented by prophylactic therapy. Repeated courses of broad spectrum antibiotics may sometimes reduce steatorrhoea in the blind loop syndrome but revision of the Polya gastrectomy may be needed.

Crohn's disease

Malabsorption in Crohn's disease can be caused by inflammation or resection of large areas of small intestinal mucosa. Bacterial proliferation in the small bowel due to stagnation caused by strictures, or enterocolic fistulae, may also be a contributory factor. An additional problem in severe Crohn's disease is inadequate dietary intake due to anorexia and increased catabolism caused by chronic inflammation. Treatment includes reducing the activity of the disease, nutritional supplementation and surgical correction of strictures and fistulae (p. 165).

Malabsorption after small bowel resection

The mechanisms causing impaired absorption following resection of jejunum or ileum have been discussed in Chapter 00.

When only a portion of the terminal ileum has been resected, the diarrhoea is usually due to spillage of bile salts into the colon, which causes the colonic mucosa to secrete rather than absorb water. Cholestyramine, which binds bile salts and makes them 'non-irritant' to the colon is, therefore, often useful in this situation. Although diarrhoea is reduced, a mild but acceptable degree of steatorrhoea may result, because binding of bile salts prevents their reabsorption which, in turn, depletes the total bile salt pool. Cholestyramine is of no use, however, in the presence of severe steatorrhoea due to more extensive resection. Under these conditions bile salts are already severely depleted because they are not being adequately reabsorbed and further loss due to binding reduces the pool below the critical level necessary for efficient fat absorption. Under these circumstances a low fat diet is advised. If this imposes an unacceptable reduction in calories or makes the diet unpalatable, medium chain triglyceride margarine and cooking oil can be used, because this type of lipid can be absorbed independently of bile salt micelles. Slowing gut transit time with codeine phosphate or loperamide often gives symptomatic relief. In rare cases, an antiperistaltic segment of small intestine has been constructed for this purpose.

In very extensive resection, liquid enteral feeding may be necessary. There are also a few patients who exist with no small intestine, being entirely dependent upon long term outpatient parenteral nutrition.

Gallstones and oxalate renal stones occur more frequently

after ileal resection because it results in disturbed bile salt and oxalate metabolism.

Small intestinal lymphoma

Both Hodgkin's and non-Hodgkin's lymphomas may occur primarily in the small bowel. The ileum is the usual site but, when complicating coeliac disease, the jejunum is commonly involved. Steatorrhoea may be the presenting problem but general malaise, pyrexia, abdominal pain and masses, profound weight loss and bleeding are also very common. Diagnosis is by small bowel barium meal, lymphangiography and laparotomy. Treatment includes resection, when possible, followed either by radiotherapy or cytotoxic drugs.

Both in the tropics and, especially, around the eastern Mediterranean, diffuse involvement of the small intestine with lymphoma is very common. There are two major categories, Mediterranean lymphoma and alpha chain disease. It seems likely that chronic malnutrition and infestation are aetiological factors. Because of the diffuse nature of these lymphomas, small bowel biopsy is frequently diagnostic. Long remission, especially in alpha chain disease, can be achieved by a combination of radiotherapy, steroids, cytotoxic drugs and antibiotics.

Chronic small bowel ischaemia

Upper abdominal colicky pain, precipitated by food, is the characteristic feature of chronic small bowel ischaemia, but diarrhoea and steatorrhoea also occur in some patients. It is very rare below the age of 50 and evidence of vascular disease elsewhere is usual. Diagnosis depends upon demonstrating stenosis or occlusion of the coeliac axis or superior mesenteric artery. The stenosed area can sometimes be bypassed with an aortomesenteric anastomosis or jump graft.

Bacterial colonization of small intestine

As already discussed (p. 83), blind loops, strictures, fistulae, diverticula and motility disturbance of the small intestine encourage bacterial proliferation. Where possible, the main aim in management is to correct the underlying anatomical abnormality surgically. An alternative approach is prolonged and repeated courses of broad spectrum antibiotics. Cholestyramine and antidiarrhoeal drugs may also be useful.

153

Post-infective malabsorption

Although not uncommon in children, bacterial infection of the gut in adults rarely gives rise to malabsorption. It is, however, more common in those who contract the disease whilst travelling overseas. The organism responsible is virtually never identified. A prolonged course of tetracycline is often needed before achieving a cure. It has been suggested that there may be a connection between this condition and tropical sprue, but the small bowel biopsy does not usually show the characteristic villous atrophy of the latter.

Giardiasis

Significant malabsorption only occasionally accompanies the diarrhoea caused by *Giardia lamblia*. The clinical features and management are discussed on p. 67.

Tropical sprue

The characteristic features of tropical sprue are malabsorption in association with widespread partial villous atrophy of the small intestine. It is found in those who inhabit or visit the tropics and occurs most frequently in south-east Asia and parts of the Caribbean. The aetiology is unknown, but it possibly results from combined nutritional deficiency and an altered microbial population of the gut. Clinical features are variable and apart from steatorrhoea and diarrhoea include megaloblastic anaemia, glossitis, pigmentation, abdominal discomfort and distension. Diagnosis depends on the appropriate history and jejunal biopsy. Many patients lose their symptoms on returning to a temperate climate. Others require long courses of treatment with folic acid and tetracycline.

Whipple's disease

In this rare disorder, malabsorption and nutritional deficiency is often preceded for many years by polyarthralgia, cough, low grade pyrexia, lymphadenopathy, abdominal discomfort and pigmentation. The small bowel biopsy is diagnostic because it reveals distended villi which contain large macrophages and dilated lymphatics. The macrophages stain heavily with periodic acid-Schiff (PAS). This PAS-positive material is bacterial glycoprotein. Electron microscopy has confirmed the presence of rod-shaped bacilli in the macrophages. Current opinion is that the disease results from a disordered immunological response to the infecting bacteria, the species of which has yet to be identified.

Pancreatic insufficiency

Pancreatic insufficiency due to chronic pancreatitis is discussed on p. 205.

16 The irritable bowel syndrome

Aetiology and pathogenesis – Clinical categories – Management

'The irritable bowel syndrome' is the term now most commonly used to describe the disorder which, in the past, has been variously called spastic colon, colonic dysfunction, hepatic and splenic flexure syndromes and mucous colitis.

The true prevalence is unknown, but it is extremely common and constitutes over 50% of referrals to most gastroenterology clinics. The ratio female:male is 2:1. Onset of symptoms is usually in the third or fourth decade. In some series a high incidence of abdominal pain and migraine in childhood has been noted.

Aetiology and pathogenesis

Psychological factors are thought to play a part in the aetiology. Several studies have shown moderate degrees of anxiety and depression in a significant proportion of patients. Many sufferers, by the time they present, have realized that stress exacerbates their disease. Nevertheless, there is a large number of patients with the irritable bowel syndrome in whom it is impossible to implicate psychogenic mechanisms. Although meals often precipitate symptoms there is usually no clear relationship to specific foods. A few patients, especially those with diarrhoea, find that milk induces their symptoms. Some of these may have coexistent alactasia. This impairs absorption of lactose by the small intestine, which has a cathartic action on entering the colon.

157

The high incidence of the irritable bowel syndrome in the developed countries has led to the suggestion that a diet low in fibre is to blame, but definite proof is lacking. Infective colitis, especially when due to amoeba, can be followed by an irritable bowel syndrome, but this is clearly of no aetiological importance in the majority of cases in Europe and North America.

Motility of the colon during an exacerbation of the irritable bowel syndrome is abnormal. Those whose main symptoms are pain and constipation have an excess of non-propulsive segmenting contractions. In those with diarrhoea there is a decrease in this type of activity. It seems likely that pain comes from distension of the bowel proximal to the area of increased segmentation. The autonomic nervous system, local neurotransmitters and hormones all have an effect upon colonic muscle activity. Recent studies suggest that patients who experience pain after meals have an abnormal colonic response to cholecystokinin which is released into the blood when food enters the duodenum. It seems that the fundamental abnormality in the irritable bowel syndrome may be a difference in the basal electrical activity of the smooth muscle when compared to normal. This, apparently, makes the colonic muscle more susceptible to nervous and humoral stimuli, which could explain why stress and meals are common exacerbating factors. Studies on the oesophagus and small intestine in patients with the irritable bowel syndrome show abnormal motility in these organs, indicating that there may be a widespread abnormality of smooth muscle function in this condition.

Clinical categories

Clinically there are three categories into which most cases of the irritable bowel syndrome can be placed.

Erratic bowel habit with pain

The largest group include those who experience pain in association with an erratic bowel habit. The pain tends to be colicky and is usually most severe in the lower abdomen. Opening the bowel or passing flatus frequently relieves this pain, but in a few patients it exacerbates their discomfort. Constipation and frequency of defaecation often alternate. The characteristic stool is pellet- or ribbon-shaped.

Postprandial pain

The next most common group comprises those in whom pain is precipitated by meals. The site is variable. When it is felt most intensely in the right or left hypochondrium the terms 'hepatic' and 'splenic' flexure syndrome are often used.

158

Painless diarrhoea

Thirdly, in approximately 10% the only symptom is diarrhoea which consists of poorly formed stool passed most frequently soon after rising.

A very common accompanying symptom in all types of the irritable bowel syndrome is a sensation of *abdominal distension*. Examination may reveal a tender left colon, but is usually unremarkable. Rectal and sigmoidoscopic examination are normal. A full blood count, erythrocyte sedimentation rate, rectal biopsy and barium enema show no abnormality.

Management

Treatment is unsatisfactory. However, *the most important point is to reassure the patient* and to emphasize particularly that their disorder has no connection with cancer or colitis. Recognition that stress is a factor can sometimes help, as may the intermittent use of mild tranquillizers, such as diazepam (Valium) and lorezepam (Ativan). Accompanying depression frequently responds to tricyclic drugs. Because of their anticholinergic activity they may also have a direct beneficial effect upon colonic smooth muscle dysfunction.

Psychological disturbance

Dietary advice and fibre

Milk or other specific foods should be avoided when symptoms are clearly related to their consumption. Increased dietary fibre is commonly prescribed and can often be dramatically successful in long term management, especially when constipation is a major problem. Unfortunately, the sensation of distension is often, at first, made worse by increased fibre. With continuing treatment this tends to improve. The initial early discomfort can often be reduced by concurrent use of antispasmodics. Because it is readily available and inexpensive, bran, two tablespoonsful daily, is the first choice. It is most conveniently taken mixed with breakfast cereals or in a small quantity of liquid. All-Bran and wholemeal bread are other acceptable means of increasing dietary fibre. Bran and its products are sometimes found unpalatable or inconvenient and, under these circumstances, one of the many proprietary products, such as Fybogel, Isogel, Normacol, Metamucil, Regulan and Prefil, should be tried.

Antispasmodic drugs

Although intravenous injections of antispasmodics relieve pain in the irritable bowel syndrome, oral anticholinergic drugs frequently prove disappointing. This is almost certainly because the dosage necessary to relax colonic muscle causes unacceptable side-effects such as dry mouth, blurred vision, bladder dysfunction and drowsiness. Nevertheless, during severe bouts of pain many patients are willing to endure these in order to obtain relief. The drugs most commonly used are propantheline (Pro-Banthine), hyoscine (Buscopan), dicyclomine (Merbentyl) and slow release atropine (Peptard). Merbeverine (Colofac) has a direct antispasmodic action on colonic smooth muscle and has no significant anticholinergic effects. It is, therefore, usually more acceptable and seems to be particularly useful taken before meals in those who suffer from postprandial pain.

Anti-
diarrhoeal
drugs

If soft, poorly formed stools are the major symptom, codeine phosphate, diphenoxylate (Lomotil) and loperamide (Imodium) will usually help. Because diarrhoea is often at its worst on rising, a regular dose at night is often beneficial.

Patients with the irritable bowel syndrome must be warned that it is a chronic remitting and relapsing condition for which, as yet, there is no cure. Present knowledge suggests they should be encouraged to persevere with a high fibre intake and use antispasmodics and antidiarrhoeal preparations when appropriate. Many will continually return to their own practitioner for reassurance, whilst others over the ensuing years will seek further numerous opinions. Repeated unnecessary investigation should be resisted.

17 Inflammatory bowel disease

Ulcerative colitis – Crohn's disease – Complications and special problems

Ulcerative colitis

Ulcerative colitis occurs most frequently in white races but is becoming more common in the developing countries of Asia and Africa. All age groups are affected. The prevalence in Britain is approximately one per 1200 of the population. There is an undoubtedly increased incidence in some families but it is not known whether the predisposition is genetic or environmental.

Aetiology and pathogenesis
The cause of ulcerative colitis is not known. It seems very likely that the disease may be due to an abnormal immunological response to either a bacterium or a virus, which has yet to be identified. The condition might then become a self-perpetuating autoimmune disorder because the immune system fails to suppress the inflammation. In the past, psychosomatic mechanisms have been implicated, but there is no good evidence to support this. The rectum is almost invariably the most severely affected area, and the condition may be confined to this area in some patients (proctitis). However, the whole large intestine is frequently involved, although the small bowel is always spared. There is a wide range in the severity of inflammation, with appearances ranging from diffuse erythema to frank ulceration and pseudopolyps. In longstanding cases, the colonic mucosa becomes pale and featureless. Fibrosis causes shortening and narrowing but, unlike Crohn's disease, strictures are rare. The histological features include a cellular infiltrate of plasma cells,

161

neutrophils and eosinophils, crypt abscesses in the mucosal glands and depletion of goblet cells. In contrast to the inflammatory reaction of Crohn's disease, the muscle and serosal layers are not involved.

Clinical features   Diarrhoea is by far the commonest symptom. Its onset may be sudden and violent but is more commonly insidious and recurrent. Several episodes may occur before presentation or diagnosis is made. Blood and mucus intimately mixed with the stool are characteristic. When the disease is restricted to the rectum, tenesmus and bleeding are the usual symptoms and true diarrhoea does not occur. Abdominal discomfort related to bowel action is common but severe pain is very unusual. Fulminant cases have fever and severe constitutional disturbance.

In patients with only proctitis there are no abnormal physical signs other than the typical sigmoidoscopic appearance of the rectum. In contrast, severe cases are frequently anaemic, dehydrated and pyrexial. *Abdominal tenderness and distension indicate severe disease.* The latter is due to dilatation of the colon, which may perforate.

Diagnosis   Diagnosis is made by sigmoidoscopy and rectal biopsy. The extent of the disease may be assessed either by barium enema or colonoscopy. All patients with proven proctitis or colitis should be instructed to seek medical attention at the first suggestion of relapse, because prompt action at this stage will frequently avert a serious exacerbation. Most gastrointestinal units now offer an urgent appointment on demand to those cases on record.

Management of proctitis   Proctitis can usually be controlled by sulphasalazine (Salazopyrin), 1 g twice daily, and local steroid preparations such as prednisolone suppositories or enemas. Once in remission, the continuance of sulphasalazine will reduce the risk of relapse. Although outpatient attendance will usually be necessary to establish the diagnosis, these patients do not require long term follow-up at hospital, providing their disease remains confined to the rectum. It should be remembered, however, that 10% will eventually develop colitis and for this group long term hospital follow-up is advisable.

Management of colitis   In acute attacks of more extensive disease, steroid enemas and sulphasalazine (Salazopyrin) are insufficient. However, providing that there are fewer than six stools per day and no systemic symptoms or excessive blood loss, admission to hospital is unnecessary. Oral prednisolone 15 mg twice daily, combined with sulphasalazine 2–3 g/d, is usually successful in such cases.

Effectiveness of treatment is judged by a reduction in stool frequency and the sigmoidoscopic appearance of the rectum. Once remission has been achieved, the dose of prednisolone should be gradually reduced and stopped after a period of 6–8 weeks. The incidence of relapse is unaffected by long term, low dose steroid therapy; such therapy, therefore, has no part to play in prophylaxis. *In contrast, sulphasalazine 1 g, twice or thrice daily, unequivocally reduces the chance of relapse and* should probably be continued indefinitely. A small number of patients are unable to take sulphasalazine because of unwanted effects. The most common is skin rash and only rarely are more serious problems, such as thrombocytopenia and anaemias, encountered. The drug may cause gastric irritation but this can usually be overcome by prescribing enteric coated tablets, reducing the dose and taking it with meals.

When sulphasalazine cannot be used, it is worth while to try azathioprine (Imuran) 100–150 mg daily. However, the efficacy of this drug in ulcerative colitis has still to be established. Codeine phosphate and loperamide give useful symptomatic relief during the first few days of a mild or moderate relapse until steroid therapy has induced remission. Long term use is rarely necessary.

Patients who in their first or subsequent attacks have *systemic disturbance, severe bleeding or more than six stools per day, should be admitted to hospital.* Inpatient care should be directed by a physician, but close consultation with a surgeon experienced in colonic surgery should be maintained throughout the initial period of treatment. These patients will have variable pyrexia, electrolyte and fluid depletion and anaemia. Treatment includes correction of the metabolic disturbance and anaemia with blood and appropriate intravenous fluids. Steroids should be administered parenterally (prednisolone 80 mg intravenously per day, or adenocorticotrophic hormone (ACTH) intramuscularly 80 units daily, or tetracosactrin acetate (Synacthen) intramuscularly, 1 mg/d). Nutrition can be maintained intravenously or by enteral tube feeding. The great majority of patients treated by this regime show a significant improvement within 5–7 d. They can then be allowed a low residue diet and parenteral steroids are replaced with oral prednisolone 40–60 mg/d. This is gradually reduced and sulphasalazine is given, as previously described, for long term prophylaxis.

Those patients who, on the above regime, show no improvement within the 5–7 days, or actually deteriorate and partic-

163

ularly if they develop toxic dilatation, are treated by urgent colectomy. Assessment during this period includes close monitoring of temperature, pulse rate, 'well-being' and the amount and frequency of stools. The abdomen should be examined at least twice daily for evidence of dilation or perforation. *It must be kept in mind that steroids may disguise the symptoms and signs of perforation and peritonitis.*

Long term follow-up

All patients with ulcerative colitis, as distinct from proctitis, should be reviewed regularly. In most situations this requires hospital follow-up. Only a small number of patients have a single attack and the usual course is one of remission and relapse. Despite the continuous use of sulphasalazine and intermittent courses of steroids, some cases cannot be controlled adequately. Colectomy must seriously be considered in these patients. Another factor that favours surgical intervention in patients with extensive colitis is recurrent active disease for more than 10 years. This group has a 30 times greater chance of developing carcinoma of the large intestine than the normal population. It is now common practice to examine these cases annually by colonoscopy. In addition to the early detection of cancer, multiple biopsies can be obtained which may show precancerous dysplastic changes. When these are found in a patient whose life is being seriously disrupted by continuing active colitis,

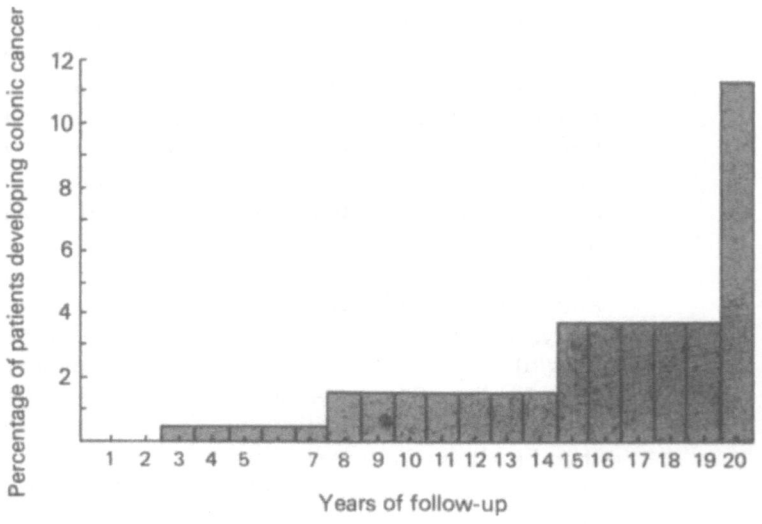

Cumulative risk in ulcerative colitis of developing colonic cancer (Radcliffe Infirmary, Oxford)

Figure 17.1

there is usually no difficulty in deciding that colectomy is necessary. However, when dysplasia is found in a patient with inactive disease, the decision is more contentious. Such patients are understandably reluctant to opt for colectomy and, as yet, it is not clear how hard they should be encouraged to do so. Patients with longstanding disease are now commonly followed-up in a 'colitis clinic' run jointly by a physician and surgeon. This makes possible the development of rapport and undoubtedly facilitates making major decisions such as the need for colectomy. Proctocolectomy is the usual operation in such cases, although many surgeons do this in two stages. The first consists of colectomy and fashioning an ileostomy. At a later stage the rectum is removed. In a minority the rectum subsequently heals sufficiently for it to be anastomosed to the ileum (ileorectal anastomosis), thus dispensing with the ileostomy. A few surgeons advocate colectomy and ileorectal anastomosis as a primary procedure. Recurrent active disease and the potential risk of cancer in the rectum are the main reasons why this operation is not more popular.

Crohn's disease

Crohn's disease, like ulcerative colitis, is most common in white races. All ages may be affected. Although the onset is most common in early adult life, presentation during adolescence seems to be increasing. Unlike the stable incidence of ulcerative colitis, that of Crohn's disease has risen during the past 20 years. It now has an approximate prevalence of 1 in 4000 in the United Kingdom. There is an increased family incidence but whether this is entirely due to genetic factors is not clear.

Aetiology and pathogenesis   The cause of Crohn's disease is unknown. Current evidence suggests that it may be due to a micro-organism. This is largely based on experiments which have shown that homogenates of bowel affected by Crohn's disease cause Crohn's-like lesions when injected into animal tissues. Furthermore, the lesion can be passaged from one animal to another. It is not known whether the putative organism is a virus or bacterium. *Acute ileitis* is commonly caused by infection with *Yersinia enterocolitica* or *Yersinia pseudotuberculosis*. However, as only a tiny number of patients with acute ileitis go on to develop chronic disease it is very unlikely that *Yersinia* is a common cause of Crohn's disease. There have been many attempts to demonstrate that patients with Crohn's disease have an impaired immunological status but results are conflicting. Nevertheless, present knowledge suggests that patients with Crohn's disease may have a disturbed immune response to antigens of varying origin that have penetrated the gut mucosa.

Unlike ulcerative colitis, the disease may involve any part of the alimentary tract from mouth to anus. The terminal ileum and caecum are most commonly affected. Lesions of the small and large intestine are often multiple and separated by mucosa of normal appearance. Although a continuous disease in the colon is not uncommon, the rectum is frequently spared, which again contrasts with the characteristic distribution in ulcerative colitis. Ulceration of the mucosa varies from superficial aphthoid lesions to deep ulcers that penetrate the submucosal layers. Adjacent loops of bowel become adherent and fistulae are common. Fibrosis is often dense, which leads to stricture formation. Histology shows transmural inflammation and fissures. In more than 50% of cases, non-caseating granulomas can be found.

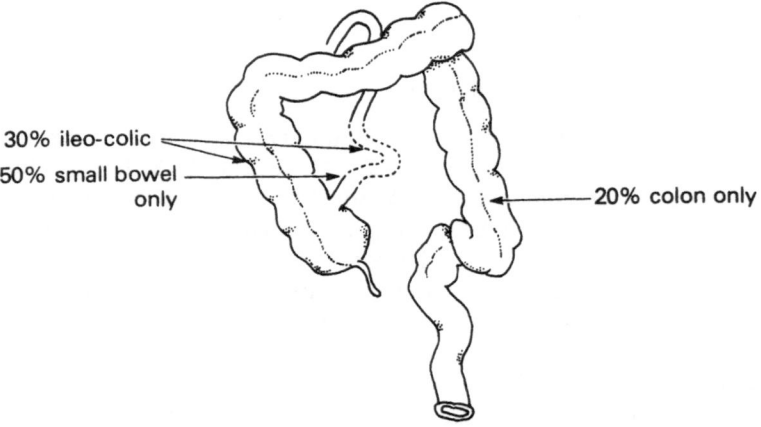

30% ileo-colic

50% small bowel only

20% colon only

Distribution of inflammation in Crohn's disease

Figure 17.2

Clinical features

The clinical features of Crohn's disease have been more fully discussed elsewhere (p. 56, 71, 84). Abdominal pain and diarrhoea are the most frequent symptoms. General malaise, weight loss and other features of malabsorption are also common. Rectal bleeding occurs, but is found less often than in ulcerative colitis. Perianal ulcers, fissures, fistulae, abscesses and fleshy skin tags surrounded by bluish-brown skin are characteristic. An abdominal mass, especially in the right iliac fossa, or signs of small bowel obstruction may occur. Nevertheless, it must be stressed that early in the course of the disease there are frequently no definite clinical features and because of this definitive diagnosis is often delayed for many years. Definitive diagnosis ultimately depends upon barium studies, sigmoidoscopy, colonoscopy or laparotomy. Barium follow-through may reveal mucosal ulceration and strictures. The barium enema in Crohn's colitis will show deep fissures and a cobblestoned appearance of the mucosa. It is also the best method of demonstrating fistulae between large and small intestine. Endoscopy of the large bowel may reveal discrete ulcers or diffuse inflammation. It is complementary to radiology in defining the distribution of the disease. *Biopsy specimens obtained by endoscopy, even when the mucosa appears macroscopically normal, may show typical submucosal inflammation.*

Medical management

Acute exacerbations of Crohn's disease should be treated with *steroids*. The regime is similar to that used in ulcerative colitis. Unfortunately the effect of steroids is often less dramatic in Crohn's disease than in ulcerative colitis and more prolonged courses are usually necessary. Pain is a prominent feature of active disease. *Antispasmodics*, such as propantheline and hyoscine (Buscopan), may be useful but more severe pain will require analgesia. Pentazocine is a useful drug in this context. Anaemia and nutritional disturbance are often severe and should be treated by transfusion and appropriate supplements. In patients with extensive small bowel disease or resection and those with enteral fistulae, tube feeding or parenteral feeding may be necessary. Intra-abdominal and perineal abscesses should be treated with antibiotics. A rational combination is co-trimoxazole (Septrin) and metronidazole (Flagyl) 200–400 mg tds.

Prophylaxis

Prevention of exacerbations is the major problem in the management of Crohn's disease. Sulphasalizine (Salazopyrine) is often used in large bowel Crohn's disease but it is certainly less effective than in ulcerative colitis. In a recent trial *azathioprine (Imuran)* was shown to reduce the relapse rate significantly, and deserves further assessment.

The place of surgery

Because surgery is eventually necessary in approximately 75% of patients with Crohn's disease, combined long term management by a physician and surgeon is advisable.

The reasons for surgery include the following.

(1) The relief of acute small bowel obstruction – although this often responds to gastric aspiration and intravenous therapy.

(2) Drainage of an abscess.

(3) Resection of gut involved in fistulae between other segments of gut, bladder, vagina and skin.

(4) Resection of a stricture that is causing recurrent bolus colic or a stagnant loop.

(5) Haemorrhage or perforation.

(6) Colitis unresponsive to medical treatment, especially when toxic dilation is threatening.

Resection of affected gut is the usual procedure and bypassing of diseased bowel is no longer favoured.

Long term follow-up   Crohn's disease is a chronic relapsing condition, but with attentive management most patients can lead a normal life. Nevertheless, the shortcomings of both medical and surgical treatment are borne out by the following facts. Patients treated medically have symptoms in 4 out of every 5 years. Of those undergoing surgical resection, more than half relapse within 10 years and many of these require a further operation. Nutritional status should be assessed at least annually. Iron, folate and vitamin B_{12} deficiency are particularly likely in those with small bowel disease or resection. Diarrhoea does not necessarily indicate reactivation of the disease and may be due to a stagnant loop or bile salt catharsis (see Chapter 7, Malabsorption). Both small and large bowel cancer are increased in Crohn's disease compared to the general population. However, the risk of developing colonic carcinoma does not appear to be as great as in ulcerative colitis.

Complications and special problems in inflammatory bowel disease

Extra-intestinal complications   Apart from the bowel complications already mentioned, both ulcerative colitis and Crohn's disease are associated with extra-intestinal problems. The frequency of these is thought to be lower in Crohn's than ulcerative colitis. The following are the most common.

Arthritis   Transient non-erosive arthritis occurs in approximately 10%, sacroileitis in 20% and ankylosing spondylitis in 5%. The activity of the arthritis usually runs parallel to that of the bowel

Skin disease   disease. A history of cutaneous vasculitis which most commonly takes the form of erythema nodosum is found in 10%, whereas pyoderma gangrenosum is much rarer. Vasculitis responds to steroid therapy but pyoderma ganrenosum is often unresponsive. In a few cases, colectomy alone is successful.

Ophthalmic disease
Conjunctivitis and uveitis often accompany arthritis and occur in about 5%. They are usually responsive to steroids. The exact aetiology of the joint, ophthalmic and cutaneous complications is unknown but they are likely to be due to circulating immune complexes that have been stimulated by gut luminal antigens crossing the diseased mucosa.

Liver disease
A wide range of liver disorders is found in inflammatory bowel disease. The association is stronger in ulcerative colitis but even in this condition chronic hepatic disease giving rise to symptoms is rare. Of these, pericholangitis is the commonest, but primary sclerosing cholangitis, chronic active hepatitis, biliary carcinoma and cirrhosis are also found. The pathogenesis of these hepatic disorders is not clear. Immune complexes again may be involved. Alternatively, bacteria or their toxins could readily cross the damaged bowel and via the portal vein pass to the liver. Colectomy, therefore, is often advised in cases of progressive liver disease.

Gallstones and renal stones
In chronic Crohn's ileitis there is an increased incidence of gallstones. This occurs because the enterohepatic circulation of bile salts is interrupted. As a consequence certain bile salts are depleted, which leads to cholesterol crystallization in the gallbladder. Oxalate absorption is increased in inflammatory bowel disease which predisposes to the formation of renal calculi. The mechanism for the increased absorption is unknown.

Disease in childhood
Diagnosis is frequently delayed in children, usually because the possibility of ulcerative colitis or Crohn's disease is not considered. Both the medical and the surgical management of acute inflammatory bowel disease in children are the same as those outlined for adults. In Crohn's disease, because courses of steroids are often more prolonged, there is a danger of stunting growth. This can be minimized by giving the steroid on alternate days or as a single morning dose.

Pregnancy
Crohn's disease or ulcerative colitis do not adversely affect established pregnancy. Because sulphasalazine has no apparent teratogenic effect it may be continued. Steroids should be used for acute exacerbations. First attacks of colitis starting in pregnancy are notoriously severe. There is no increased rate of relapse during pregnancy in either condition but the puerperium is often associated with an exacerbation.

18 Diverticular disease of the colon

Diffuse diverticulosis – Sigmoid diverticulosis

The two commonest forms of diverticular disease of the colon are diffuse diverticulosis and sigmoid diverticulosis.

Diffuse diverticulosis

As the name 'diffuse diverticulosis' implies, diverticula are found throughout the colon. The colon tends to be atrophic and dilated and the diverticula are shallow with wide apertures. The aetiology is unknown but, because in the United Kingdom one third of the population over 60 have these lesions, it is considered to be a degenerative process.

There is no specific treatment but, as *constipation* is a common symptom, fibre-based laxatives are usually prescribed. Apart from constipation, diffuse diverticulosis may present with *bleeding per rectum*. Severity varies but the majority of patients are treated successfully with bed rest and transfusion. If bleeding continues resection may be necessary. Angiography is the most accurate means of identifying the bleeding site. *Perforation* is the other major complication and usually leads to generalized peritonitis. Treatment is by laparotomy and peritoneal cleansing. Local repair of the perforation may be possible, but frequently it is neccesary to exteriorize or resect the involved segment and fashion a proximal colostomy.

Sigmoid diverticulosis

When mainly localized to the sigmoid colon, diverticula are thought to result from increased intracolonic pressures in that

171

region. This is associated with muscular hypertrophy, unco-ordinated contractions and reduction of the colonic lumen. The diverticula tend to be long and have narrow necks. Because the condition is extremely rare in societies that take a high roughage diet, it has been argued that a refined Western diet is causative. Presentation is unusual before the age of 50. Early symptoms are probably due to the uncoordinated colonic function and include *vague abdominal discomfort, distension* and *small fragmented stools.* On examination, there is frequently no abnormality although it may be possible to palpate a slightly tender sigmoid colon. With increasing hypertrophy of colonic muscle the patient experiences *colicky pain,* and *large bowel obstruction* may eventually occur. Diagnosis is confirmed by barium enema.

Diverticulitis

Stasis in a diverticulum predisposes to *inflammation.* The term 'diverticulitis' should be reserved for this condition. Pyrexia, malaise and lower abdominal pain are the major symptoms. Examination reveals definite tenderness and guarding. An inflamed diverticulum may *perforate,* causing a localized *pericolic abscess.* On rectal examination it is often possible to palpate a tender extrinsic mass. Generalized *faecal peritonitis* following perforation is relatively rare. Spread of infection to the bladder gives rise to *frequency of micturition* and *dysuria.* This may progress to a vesico-colic *fistula* giving rise to pneumaturia. Fistulae may also develop between the colon and vagina causing *vaginal discharge.* A fistulous tract between large and small intestine, although relatively rare, may cause a *stagnant loop syndrome* and *malabsorption* (p. 83).

Management

The symptoms of *uncomplicated sigmoid diverticular disease* are usually relieved by a high fibre regime. This may be in the form of natural bran (30 ml daily), bran tablets (Fybranta, Proctofibe) or All-Bran. If symptoms continue, non-bran fibre should be added to the regime (Fybogel, Normacol, Prefil, Metamucil). Many patients complain that increased dietary fibre causes increased flatulence and distension. They must be reassured that this is a temporary effect and that it will improve with time. The problem can often be alleviated by starting with small amounts of fibre and gradually increasing the quantities until the maximum benefit has been achieved. Mebeverine (Colofac) seems to reduce the sensation of distension during this initial phase. It is also useful, together with anticholinergic drugs (Pro-Banthine, Buscopan, Peptard, Cantil) for the relief of colicky pain. *The patient must be strongly reassured that he or she does not have cancer.*

When there is evidence of inflammation, a broad spectrum antibiotic, such as Amoxil or Septrin, should be given until the inflammation has resolved. A fluid diet is given during this period, together with regular analgesics such as pentazocine (Fortral). Opiates and codeine must be avoided because they cause colonic contraction and increased intraluminal pressures. Most patients can be treated at home but if there is no significant improvement within 48 h, then admission to hospital is advisable.

Surgery   A poor response or worsening condition may be due to intestinal obstruction, perforation or abscess. Surgery is usually indicated in such cases. Primary excision of the diseased segment may be possible. This is usually combined with a temporary colostomy, re-anastomosis being left to a second operation. In many cases excision is not possible and all that can be offered is peritoneal toilet and a transverse colostomy. The diseased segment is subsequently resected when the inflammation has settled and the patient's condition has improved.

Fistulae   Resection will also be necessary if a fistula has formed and in those experiencing recurrent severe inflammatory exacerbations.

Elective surgery   The place of elective surgery in non-inflammatory diverticular disease is not clear. Some surgeons will resect a severely hypertrophied section of the sigmoid colon when this is causing

Sigmoid myotomy   bouts of severe colic. An alternative to resection is sigmoid myotomy. In this operation the circular colonic muscle is divided longitudinally. Although this lowers intraluminal pressures, symptoms often return 2–3 years later.

173

19 Common liver diseases

Viral Hepatitis

Hepatitis type A – Hepatitis type B – Hepatitis type non-A, non-B – Complications of hepatitis

Three distinct categories of viral hepatitis are now recognized. The viruses responsible are type A, type B and type non-A, non-B.

Hepatitis type A

The virus causing this disease can be isolated from the faeces of patients during the incubation and early symptomatic phase of the illness. The electron microscope shows that it is a particle 24–29 nm in size.

The usual means of transmission is the faecal–oral route. The incubation period is 15–50 d. There is usually person-to-person contact, but contamination of food and water may also be responsible. Shellfish are a common source of hepatitis A virus. The disease is most common in underdeveloped countries. A carrier state does not appear to exist. Recent studies suggest that subclinical anicteric hepatitis type A is very common and that it is these cases that maintain the virus in the population.

Clinical features
Severity of type A hepatitis is variable but in general the disease is less serious than type B infection. Many patients, probably the majority, do not become jaundiced. Their predominant symptoms are anorexia, malaise, mild fever and gastrointestinal disturbance. In those who become icteric, symptoms usually antedate jaundice by 3–10 d. The liver is enlarged and tender and the spleen is sometimes palpable. The patient may

175

notice dark urine and pale stools a few days before jaundice becomes obvious. The onset of jaundice is often rapidly followed by remission of malaise.

In the majority, jaundice clears within a month, although lethargy may persist for several more weeks. Relapse sometimes occurs but is usually mild and shortlived. During the acute phase of the illness, even when the patient is anicteric, serum aminotransferases are greatly elevated. Serum bilirubin levels are variably increased and the alkaline phosphatase may also be mildly raised. Antibodies against hepatitis virus type A are found in the serum throughout the acute phase of illness and are detectable for many years. Immunity is probably lifelong.

Management

Admission to hospital is not necessary in most cases. The patient usually confines himself to bed during the first few days but as soon as he begins to improve strict bed rest is not essential. Barrier nursing is unnecessary, but the patient must exercise special care with the disposal of excreta and washing of hands for at least a week after the appearance of jaundice. Use of a separate lavatory is ideal. A free diet should be allowed. Drugs, including corticosteroids, are of no proven benefit in the routine management of acute viral hepatitis. *Six months abstinence from alcohol is obligatory.* A warning should be given that failure to do so will precipitate relapse.

Admission to hospital

Admission to hospital is usually for social reasons which include unsatisfactory toilet arrangements, absence of someone to look after the patient or the presence of infants in the house. The other major reason for admission is the severity of disease (see below, p. 178, fulminant hepatitis).

Prevention

Travellers to countries with a high incidence of hepatitis may be protected for 2 months by a prophylactic intramuscular injection of human γ-globulin. It is also effective in preventing the disease in contacts of hepatitis patients when given within 2 weeks of exposure.

Hepatitis type B

The virus causing this disease is the 42 nm 'Dane particle'. Antigens from this virus, one of which is called 'Australia antigen', can be detected in the serum of patients before and during the acute phase of the illness.

Transmission may occur by the parenteral or non-parenteral route. In the past, infection rates were high in patients requiring multiple transfusions, such as those with bleeding conditions and those receiving haemodialysis. Screening of blood donors for hepatitis B antigen has now reduced the spread via blood and its products. Nevertheless, an increased incidence is found in drug addicts sharing needles, and also in laboratory staff dealing with contaminated blood. Venereal transmission is common and particularly so in male homosexuals. The incubation period is from 6 weeks to 6 months.

The discovery of virus antigens has made possible the identification of chronic carriers of hepatitis B virus. The majority of carriers are healthy and are only discovered by routine screening of blood. The risk of contracting the disease from these subjects is probably very small. Some chronic carriers of hepatitis B antigens go on to develop chronic active hepatitis, cirrhosis or hepatoma.

Clinical features
Symptoms and signs are the same as those of hepatitis type A. There is a similar wide range in the severity of illness; however, the prodromal period is often longer and constitutional disturbance greater. The risk of a fulminant course and fatal outcome is also greater. Rashes, arthritis and circulating immune complexes are additional characteristic features of type B infection.

Polyarteritis
In some instances infection with type B virus appears to induce a chronic polyarteritis and polyarthritis.

Management
The principles of management are the same as those for hepatitis A and admission to hospital is governed by the same factors.

Prevention
A specific anti-hepatitis B immunoglobulin is available. When contaminated material is accidentally introduced, either by splashing onto mucous membranes or by pricking, the specific immunoglobulin should be administered as soon as possible and repeated at 4 weeks. *The sexual partners of patients should also be offered prophylaxis.* It is likely that vaccination against hepatitis B virus will soon be available.

Hepatitis type non-A, non-B

This agent appears to be an important cause of hepatitis transmitted by blood products, although it can also be spread by the non-parenteral route. The incubation period varies from 5 weeks to 5 months. It is a probable cause of chronic liver disease.

Complications of hepatitis

Acute viral hepatitis may be complicated by the development of fulminant hepatitis, prolonged cholestasis, chronic hepatitis, cirrhosis and hepatoma.

Fulminant
hepatitis

Fortunately, fulminant hepatitis is very rare. In a few cases of rapidly progressive hepatitis, the patient's condition deteriorates before the jaundice has fully developed. More commonly, a fulminant course is accompanied by deepening jaundice. Other ominous features are vomiting, bruising and signs of encephalopathy, including a flapping tremor, confusion, stupor or coma.

Prolonged
cholestasis

In a minority of patients, jaundice fails to resolve within the usual 4–6 weeks, despite an obvious general improvement. Itching becomes troublesome and the liver function tests have a cholestatic pattern with greatly elevated levels of alkaline phosphatase and a comparatively small rise in the transaminases. The condition must be distinguished from extrahepatic biliary obstruction and drug jaundice (p. 182). The condition resolves clinically and histologically within 6 months.

Chronic
hepatitis

Chronic hepatitis can be defined as inflammation of the liver which continues for more than 6 months without evidence of resolution. It is a sequel to type B and probably type non-A, non-B infection. There are two categories – chronic persistent and chronic active hepatitis. The former is non-progressive and complete recovery is usual, although this may take several years. In contrast, chronic active hepatitis is characterized by continuing liver damage which may eventually lead to cirrhosis (see below).

Cirrhosis

The discovery of serological markers for hepatitis B infection has confirmed that infection with this virus may, in a small proportion of patients, progress to cirrhosis (see below).

Hepatoma

There is a high incidence of primary hepatocellular cancer in areas of the world where hepatitis B infection is common. Although cirrhosis and hepatoma are closely associated, the former is not always present in patients with type B serological markers and hepatoma, which suggests that the virus may be directly oncogenic.

Chronic Hepatitis

Chronic persistent hepatitis – Chronic active hepatitis

Chronic hepatitis can be defined as inflammation of the liver which continues for more than 6 months without evidence of resolution. Two distinct categories, largely based upon histological features, are recognized. They are (1) chronic persistent hepatitis and (2) chronic active hepatitis.

Chronic persistent hepatitis

The histological characteristics of chronic persistent hepatitis are mononuclear cell infiltration of the portal tracts, preservation of normal lobular structure and absence of 'piecemeal' necrosis.

Although many causes of chronic persistent hepatitis have been identified, the aetiology is obscure in many cases. *Hepatitis types B* and *non-A,non-B* may persist for more than 6 months. An acute *alcoholic hepatitis* may progress in similar fashion. *Ulcerative colitis, Crohn's* and *coeliac disease* may also be associated with these histological features in the liver. *Drugs*, including paracetamol, aspirin, methyldopa, isoniazid and some cytotoxic agents are capable of inducing a persistent hepatic inflammatory reaction.

Clinical features When hepatitis B virus is responsible, there may be failure to make a complete recovery from the acute attack with continuing lethargy, hepatic tenderness and intolerance to alcohol. Some patients, especially with other aetiologies, present with these symptoms without any noticeable acute phase. Yet others are asymptomatic, the disease only being discovered because of blood testing for other reasons. The typical physical signs of chronic liver disease, such as spider naevi, liver palms and fluid retention, are absent.

Investigation Serum transaminase concentrations are markedly raised, but bilirubin, alkaline phosphatase and protein levels are normal. Liver biopsy is necessary to distinguish the condition from chronic active hepatitis.

Management There is no specific treatment and steroids are not indicated. Prolonged abstinence from alcohol is essential. Although the patient must be warned that recovery may take several years, he should be strongly reassured that it will be complete and that cirrhosis will not develop.

Chronic active hepatitis

The histological characteristics of this condition are lymphocyte and plasma cell infiltration of the portal tracts, disruption of the liver lobule with 'piecemeal' necrosis and extensive fibrosis.

As with chronic persistent hepatitis, *types B* and *non-A,* non-B *viruses, alcohol* and *drugs* (oxyphenisatin, methyldopa, isoniazid) are known aetiological agents. The majority of cases have no known cause. Within this latter group are those patients with *lupoid hepatitis.* When chronic active hepatitis occurs in children or adolescents, *Wilson's disease* must also be considered. This condition results from a metabolic defect which leads to copper deposition in body tissues. The areas most severely affected are the basal ganglia and liver. It is an inherited condition and the mode of transmission is autosomal recessive. Consanguinity of parents is found in more than 50% of cases. The pathogenic processes in chronic active hepatitis are not understood but it has been suggested that viruses, drugs, alcohol and probably other agents initiate liver damage. This releases or changes the antigenicity of liver tissue which, in turn, stimulates an autoimmune process. Clones of lymphocytes sensitized in this way then continue to damage the liver in the absence of the initiating agent. It seems likely that affected subjects have a genetic predisposition to mount inappropriate immune reactions.

Hepatitis B group   Chronic active hepatitis associated with hepatitis B virus affects males more frequently than females and has an increased incidence in groups at particular risk to hepatitis type B (p. 177). Patients with impaired immunological function, such as those with malignancy and those taking immunosuppressive drugs, are also more likely to develop the disease. Onset is usually in the third to fifth decade. The clinical presentations are similar to those of chronic persistent hepatitis.

Lupoid group   In the lupoid type there is a female:male predominance of 3:1. Onset tends to be in adolescence or during the fifth decade. Presentation may be acute, resembling viral hepatitis, with subsequent failure to resolve. Other patients have a more insidious onset with lethargy and general malaise. Spider naevi and seborrhoeic rashes are early signs. Recurrent episodes of jaundice are common, and as the disease progresses other signs of chronic liver failure occur. It is in the lupoid type of chronic hepatitis that autoimmune processes are most prominent and the condition is often associated with other immunopathic disorders. These include autoimmune thyroid disease, ulcerative colitis, polyarthritis, fibrosing alveolitis and the sicca syndrome. Endocrine disturbance is common and includes diabetes mellitus, Cushingoid features, amenorrhoea in females and gynaecomastia in males.

Investigation   Serum levels of bilirubin and transaminases are variably raised and may fluctuate widely. There is an increase in the γ-globulin fraction of the serum proteins and frequently a reduction in albumin. The IgG level is particularly high in lupoid hepatitis. Antigens derived from hepatitis B virus are found in chronic active hepatitis due to this virus but not in lupoid hepatitis. In contrast, smooth muscle antibodies in high titre are found in 60% of lupoid cases but not in hepatitis B related disease. Antinuclear antibody occurs in 50%, LE cells in 15% and mitochondrial antibody in 25% of patients with lupoid hepatitis.

When the disorder presents in adolescents or young adults, Wilson's disease must be excluded by slit lamp examination of the cornea for Kayser–Fleischer rings, measuring levels of serum copper and caeruloplasmin and the copper content of liver biopsy tissue.

Course and management

Drug induced disease

The offending drug must be withdrawn and should not be reintroduced. Under these circumstances the disease is not progressive and prognosis is good.

Wilson's disease

Continuing liver damage can be arrested by early treatment with the chelating agent, penicillamine. Prognosis is comparatively good in those treated before neurological symptoms have appeared. Untreated, the liver lesion progresses. The common causes of death are hepatocellular failure, haemorrhage from varices or one of the complications of severe neurological deficit.

Lupoid hepatitis

Prenisolone 10–15 mg daily leads to clinical, biochemical and histological improvement in a large proportion of patients and early mortality is reduced. Treatment should continue for at least 6 months, and may be needed for several years in some cases. Azathioprine 50 mg daily is sometimes added to the prednisolone regime, particularly in those who fail to respond to the steroid alone. The natural progression of the liver lesion is to cirrhosis. Without treatment there is a 60% mortality within 5 years of onset, from either liver failure or bleeding varices. The effect of treatment on long term survival is not yet clear.

Virus type B chronic active hepatitis

The value of prednisolone and azathioprine in this group has yet to be proved. However, in patients with significant symptoms, Sherlock suggests a 6-month trial of prednisolone 10–20 mg daily, the benefit being assessed clinically, biochemically and histologically. If there is no obvious improvement, it is unlikely that a more prolonged course will be useful. In patients with only minor symptoms, steroid therapy is probably not indicated. However, if rebiopsy at 6 months indicates progression of the hepatic lesion, it seems reasonable to give a trial course of prednisolone. In general, this type of chronic active hepatitis progresses towards cirrhosis more slowly than lupoid hepatitis. There is, however, an increased incidence of primary liver cancer.

Drug induced liver disease

Direct hepatotoxicity – Toxicity due to drug metabolites – 'Hypersensitivity' induced damage – Halothane – Canalicular cholestasis – Other hepatic reactions to drugs

Although knowledge about drug induced liver damage has advanced in recent years, the exact pathogenic mechanisms in many instances are not clearly understood and, as yet, there is no definitive classification of hepatic complications of drug therapy. The most satisfactory so far proposed is that of Sherlock.

Direct hepatotoxicity

Tetracyclines are the only widely used group of therapeutic agents that directly cause damage to hepatocytes. The degree of injury is related to blood levels. Therefore high dosages, especially when given intravenously, are particularly likely to cause damage. Impaired renal function increases the risk. The major toxic effect on the liver is interference with protein synthesis. Because this function is also normally reduced in late pregnancy and malnutrition, tetracyclines should not be used in these situations. Serum transaminase and urine urobilinogen concentrations rise, but bilirubin levels are often only slightly increased. The prothrombin time is prolonged due to reduced clotting factor synthesis. The liver becomes fatty because production of lipid transporting protein is also affected.

Cytotoxic drugs used in the treatment of cancer and leukaemia may also cause hepatic damage by a direct action. These include mithramicine, mitomycin and actinomycin D.

Toxicity due to drug metabolites

The liver is the major site of drug metabolism. Many drugs although non-toxic themselves are converted into hepatotoxic metabolites by liver enzyme systems. This takes place in both the microsomes and the cytosol of hepatocytes. The main microsomal enzymes responsible for this process are dinucleotide phosphate C reductase and cytochrome P 450. An increase in these enzymes is induced by other drugs such as phenobarbitone and alcohol. Thus patients who have been taking these substances are likely to produce greater quantities of toxic metabolites more rapidly, and are therefore more susceptible.

Paracetamol   Poisoning with *paracetamol* is now the commonest example of injury due to toxic metabolites. Under normal circumstances, the toxic metabolite of paracetamol is removed by conjugation with glutathione. However, hepatic stores of glutathione are limited, and become exhausted when more than 15–20 g of paracetamol are suddenly ingested. Most fatalities occur following the ingestion of about 40 g of paracetamol. The toxic metabolite causes centizonal necrosis of liver lobules and, in severe cases, total disruption of liver structure and function. The initial symptoms of poisoning are anorexia and vomiting which come on within a few hours. These rapidly resolve, but in those with significant liver damage jaundice, liver tenderness and a bleeding tendency develop during the third and fourth days. The majority of patients make a steady recovery after this and cirrhosis is not a subsequent complication. In contrast, others go into fatal fulminant hepatic failure with coma and renal failure.

Treatment consists of gastric lavage followed by the early administration of cysteamine. This substance is a precursor of glutathione and therefore promotes synthesis of the latter. The regular long term use of paracetamol has been implicated in a small number of patients with chronic hepatitis.

Carbon tetrachloride   Toxic metabolite production is the mechanism of carbon tetrachloride liver damage and is probably involved in the hepatotoxicity of other aromatic solvents. The characteristic features are jaundice within 48 h, hepatic tenderness, gastritis, spontaneous bleeding, renal failure and drowsiness. Cirrhosis does not occur in those who recover.

183

Isoniazid   The antituberculous drug, isoniazid, after acetylation is converted in the liver to a toxic metabolite. A subgroup of the population rapidly acetylate isoniazid, and these individuals have a greater chance of developing isoniazid toxicity. The combination of isoniazid with rifampicin also increases the chance of liver damage. This is probably because rifampicin induces microsomal enzymes and therefore enhances the formation of toxic metabolites from the isoniazid. Toxicity is more common in those over 35, but the reason for this is not clear. Histologically there may be centrizonal necrosis, but in other cases changes similar to viral hepatitis are seen. The disorder usually has an insidious onset, coming on several weeks or months after the start of treatment. Anorexia and lethargy are common early complaints, followed by jaundice. Monitoring of isoniazid therapy by regular liver function tests is advisable. The drug should be stopped if there is a persistent rise in transaminase levels or clinical evidence of hepatic damage.

Methyldopa   The mechanism of methyldopa (Aldomet) hepatotoxicity is not entirely clear but metabolites seem to be involved. Symptoms suggestive of viral hepatitis, including jaundice, predominate. They usually develop between 1 and 4 months after commencing treatment. Most patients are not severely affected, but fulminant hepatic failure sometimes occurs. Chronic active hepatitis and even cirrhosis may develop if the drug is not withdrawn.

Oxyphenisatin   In the past, a similar clinical spectrum was seen in long term users of oxyphenisatin-containing laxatives. This drug has now been withdrawn in most parts of the world, but is still available in a few European countries. It is also a constituent of some laxatives sold in 'health' stores.

Methotrexate   The folic acid competitor, methotrexate, is a valuable drug in the treatment of severe psoriasis. Unfortunately, one of its metabolites induces hepatic fibrosis and in some cases cirrhosis. Toxicity is associated with long term usage. Methotrexate therapy should, therefore, be monitored by serial liver biopsies and be withdrawn if fibrosis occurs.

'Hypersensitivity' induced damage

Although in many cases of metabolite induced hepatic damage a direct effect of the metabolite on hepatocytes seems probable, it remains possible that in some cases 'hypersensitivity' reactions against the liver could be induced by the drug or a metabolite combining with hepatic tissue, thus converting it into an antigen.

Humoral and cell mediated immunological reactions would then be stimulated and bring about liver cell damage. A large group of drugs are considered to cause liver damage by this mechanism. In some, the predominant feature is cholestasis, whereas others cause a more generalized hepatocellular dysfunction.

The characteristics of hypersensitivity reactions are that:

(1) Only a small number of those taking the drug are affected.
(2) Arthralgia, fever, rashes and eosinophilia are common.
(3) There is no relationship to dose.
(4) They are more common after multiple exposure.

Chlor-promazine

Chlorpromazine (Largactil) and, less commonly, other promazine derivatives cause a hypersensitivity cholestatic jaundice. This usually comes on between 1 and 4 weeks after start of treatment and is often preceded by a few days of malaise and anorexia. Serum transaminases may be moderately raised, but the striking biochemical feature is the great elevation of alkaline phosphatase. Symptoms and jaundice usually resolve rapidly without sequelae, once the drug has been withdrawn. Persistence beyond 3 months is uncommon, but a few patients have remained jaundiced for over 2 years. In such cases, ultrasound scanning of the liver will distinguish the condition from extrahepatic obstructive jaundice and liver biopsy will exclude primary biliary cirrhosis.

Chlor-propamide
Azathioprine
Erythromycin estolate

The hypoglycaemic drug chlorpropamide (Diabinese), and the immunosuppressant agent, azathioprine (Imuran), may also cause a similar cholestatic jaundice.

The estolate formulation of erythromycin, but not erythromycin stearate, causes a hypersensitivity reaction which usually results in cholestatic jaundice. Abdominal pain and fever are common accompanying symptoms.

Nitrofurantoin
Carbimazole

The antibacterial nitrofurantoin (Furadantin) and the antithyroidal drug, carbimazole (Neo-Mercazol), may very rarely cause a hypersensitivity reaction in the liver. With these drugs there is a more generalized hepatocyte dysfunction resembling hepatitis, in contrast to the almost pure cholestatic type of reaction seen with the promazines.

Many other drugs induce generalized hypersensitivity reactions affecting many different organs and tissues. Most give rise to a 'hepatitis' and present within 6 weeks of starting the drug. Para-aminosalicylate (PAS), sulphonamides, phenindione (Dindevan), diphenylhydantoin and phenylbutazone (Butazolidin) have been implicated in such reactions.

Halothane

A single exposure to the anaesthetic agent, halothane, is very rarely associated with liver damage. Halothane 'hepatitis' is most common after repeated use of the gas. The initial symptoms are pyrexia and general malaise which come on between 1 and 2 weeks after the operation. Jaundice follows a few days later. Histology reveals centrizonal necrosis and infiltration of the sinusoids with leukocytes. Granulomas are common, and the repair phase is characterized by large amounts of collagen deposition. There is often a peripheral blood eosinophilia. The degree of icterus is variable. In those with significant clinical jaundice, there is a 20% mortality. The mechanism of halothane hepatitis is still unclear. However, the delayed onset, increased incidence following multiple exposure, pyrexia, eosinophilia and granulomas, point to a hypersensitivity reaction.

Canalicular cholestasis

Canalicular cholestasis is not due to hypersensitivity and there is no inflammatory reaction in the liver. The histology shows only cholestasis. The mechanism is not clear, but a direct toxic effect on canalicular and Golgi apparatus membrane or disturbance of bile salt micelle production are strong possibilities. The agents that cause these reactions are the 17-α-alkylated steroids such as methyltestosterone (Perandren), and anabolic compounds such as norethandrolone (Nilevar), methandienone (Dianabol) and oxymetholone (Anapolon). The oestrogen analogues of many contraceptive pills also contain 17-alkalated compounds capable of causing cholestasis. The severity of reaction to these substances is dose related, although some patients appear to be genetically susceptible to very small amounts. This is probably the explanation for the cholestasis seen in a small number of women taking the pill. These are the same subjects who also suffer from cholestatic symptoms during late pregnancy. The earliest symptom of this type of cholestasis is generalized pruritis due to bile salt retention, and jaundice usually develops only if the drug is continued or the dose increased. Withdrawal of the preparation is followed by complete recovery.

Other hepatic reactions to drugs

Oestrogen increases the concentration of cholesterol in bile and, predictably, women who have taken contraceptive pills

Gallstones have an increased incidence of gallstones.

Chronic The role of drugs in chronic hepatitis is discussed else-
hepatitis where (p. 180).

Hepatomas *Benign adenomas* of the liver occur with increased frequency in women taking the contraceptive pill, although the actual risk is very small. The characteristic presentation is right hypochondrial pain or a mass in the liver. These tumours are highly vascular and have a tendency to bleed into either the hepatic tissue or the peritoneum. The diagnosis is confirmed by radionuclide and ultrasound scanning or angiography. Biopsy should not be attempted because of the danger of haemorrhage. Resection of the tumour is the treatment of choice.

Hepatocellular carcinoma has an increased incidence in women taking contraceptives. However, the numbers are even smaller than for benign hepatoma. There is also an association between hepatocellular carcinoma and the 17-alkalated anabolic steroids.

Alcoholic liver disease

Disease of the liver due to alcohol can be divided into three main categories – fatty deposition, inflammatory infiltration and cirrhosis. The exact incidence of alcoholic liver disease is not known, but it seems likely that the number with alcoholic cirrhosis represents only one third of the total. Two thirds of all cases of cirrhosis in England and Wales are now due to alcohol, and in the United States of America it causes more than 20 000 deaths per annum. Throughout the world there is a direct relationship between alcohol consumption per capita and the death rate from cirrhosis. The highest incidence is seen in the wine-producing countries of Western Europe. In Britain, cirrhosis is most common in company directors, licensees, barmen, entertainers, seamen, the armed forces and doctors.

Pathogenesis Ethyl alcohol disturbs lipid and carbohydrate metabolism in the liver, and taken in excess leads to *fat deposition* within hepatocytes, which is termed '*steatosis*'. In certain individuals, excessive amounts of alcohol have a direct cytopathic effect upon hepatocytes. This cell death stimulates an inflammatory reaction and these changes constitute *alcoholic hepatitis*. The typical feature of alcoholic hepatitis is focal necrosis of hepatocytes particularly in the centrilobular areas. Polymorphs rather than mononuclear cells often predominate. Fibrosis

Table 19.1 Risk of death from cirrhosis by occupation (average risk = 1)

Publicans	15
Seamen	8
Hotel and catering	5
Financiers	4
Journalists	3
Doctors	3
Judges and lawyers	2
Doctors' wives	2

around the central veins and Mallory's hyaline material within hepatocytes are also commonly seen. In some cases, fibrosis is especially intense and collagen bands form bridges between the portal and the central areas of lobules. This is frequently accompanied by disorganized nodular regeneration of liver tissue. These two features constitute *cirrhosis*. The nodules in alcoholic cirrhosis are usually small and this category is termed 'micronodular'. Larger nodules may, however, occur and it is in this 'macronodular' type that a primary hepatoma most frequently arises. Why some individuals never develop cirrhosis, despite consuming large quantities of alcohol, is not known. It does not appear to be related to particular types of alcoholic drinks or to coexistent malnutrition. It seems more likely that a subgroup of alcohol abusers have a genetic predisposition to alcoholic hepatitis and cirrhosis which, in turn, may have an immunopathic basis. It has been suggested that a coexistent virus infection could be a factor. A continuously excessive intake is more commonly associated with cirrhosis than are recurrent binges – perhaps because the latter pattern allows hepatocytes to 'recuperate' between insults.

Clinical features
The patient with alcoholic liver disease may present because of:

(1) Non-hepatic alcohol related problems (depression, loss of libido, fits, drunken driving, violence)
(2) Routine or insurance examination
(3) Hepatopathic symptoms.

A common group of symptoms in alcohol abusers is morning nausea and retching, accompanied by a tendency to pass loose stool. Retching often produces small haematemases due to oesophageal tearing. Such patients also have an increased incidence of gastric erosions and duodenal ulcer which are additional causes of dyspepsia and gastrointestinal bleeding. These relatively mild symptoms are usually associated with steatosis, and frequently the only abnormal physical sign is moderate hepatomegaly. A similar spectrum of symptoms occurs in alcoholic hepatitis, but they are usually more severe. Acute exacerbations of alcoholic hepatitis are frequently precipitated by bouts of heavy drinking or incidental infections. Pyrexia, sweats, jaundice, vomiting, diarrhoea and pain in the right hypochondrium are the major features of these acute phases. Examination reveals a tender enlarged liver and, in some patients, ascites. Other signs of liver failure, such as palmar erythema, spider naevi, testicular atrophy, gynaeco-mastia and bruising are also very common. Neuropsychiatric disturbance may be due to the alcoholism *per se* or hepato-cellular failure.

By the time alcoholic liver disease has progressed to cirrhosis, one or more of the above clinical signs is almost invariably present. Fluid retention with ascites and ankle oedema is particularly common. Portal hypertension causes splenomegaly and gastro-oesophageal varices. Bleeding from the latter is a frequent cause of death. Dupuytren's contracture and parotid swelling are additional signs that point to an alcoholic aetiology.

Investigation

Tests of liver function may show normal results in *steatosis*, although there is usually an elevation of the serum γ-glutamyl-transpeptidase and transaminases. Red cell macrocytosis should always raise the suspicion of alcohol abuse.

Alcoholic hepatitis is associated with variably raised serum levels of bilirubin, alkaline phosphatase, γ-glutamyl-transpeptidase and transaminases. Plasma albumin is low and γ-globulin increased. Hyperlipaemia is often found and is some-times accompanied by red cell haemolysis. Polymorpholeuko-cytosis, which is present in acute alcoholic hepatitis, helps to distinguish it from viral hepatitis, in which the white cell count is either normal or shows a lymphocytosis.

The serum bilirubin, enzyme and protein abnormalities are also found in *cirrhosis*, although in well-compensated patients they may be normal or only marginally disturbed. Liver biopsy is the only definite means of diagnosing which category of alcoholic liver disease is present, and should be performed whenever blood coagulative function and platelet count permit. A prothrombin time not more than 3 seconds prolonged compared with the control and a platelet count of more than 80 000/mm^3 are the acceptable parameters.

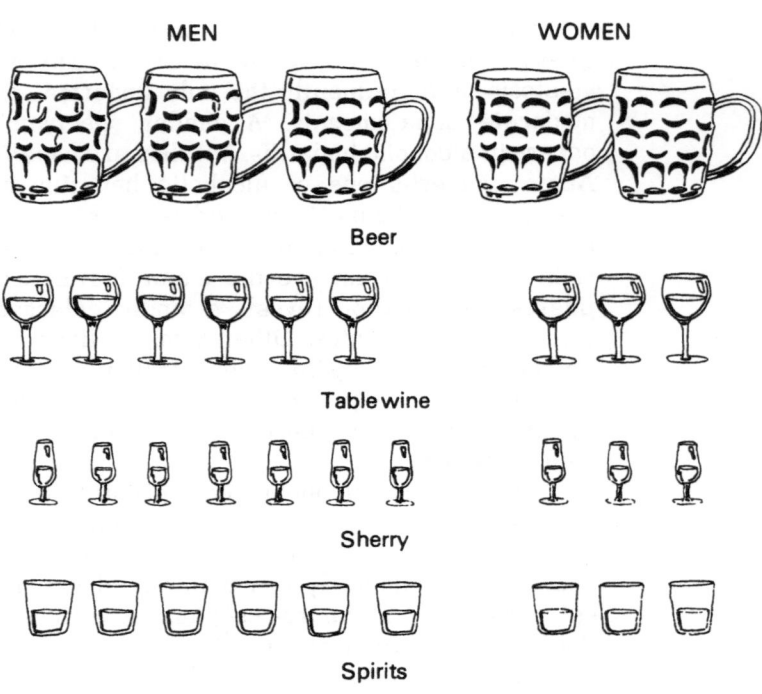

MEN   WOMEN

Beer

Table wine

Sherry

Spirits

Proposed 'safe' daily limits of alcohol consumption

Figure 19.1

Management   In patients whose biopsies show only fatty deposition, and in whom there is no psychological dependence on alcohol, total abstinence is unnecessary. Provided that such patients keep consumption within reasonable limits, they are unlikely to develop more severe forms of alcoholic liver disease. It is impossible to be dogmatic about what is a 'reasonable' amount of alcohol, but two facts should be kept in mind. The first is that women have a far greater risk of developing severe alcoholic liver disease and their 'safe amount' is less than for men. The second is that for men the daily consumption over a 10-year period of one third of a bottle of spirits or one bottle of table wine, or two thirds of a bottle of sherry or 5–6 pints of beer is associated with a high risk of alcoholic cirrhosis. Obviously, patients must be instructed to keep well below these levels. Avoiding lunchtime drinking and restricting consumption to the evening will often force a heavy drinker into more acceptable and healthy habits.

In patients dependent upon alcohol, regardless of the

degree of liver pathology, and in those with hepatitis, total abstinence is essential. This is necessary because there is overwhelming evidence that alcoholic hepatitis is a pre-cirrhotic condition. In cirrhosis the position is less clear, but it seems likely that total abstinence does significantly prolong life, especially in those patients who have not already suffered from variceal haemorrhage. Alcohol dependence should be dealt with along the usual lines. Psychiatrists, social workers and self-help organizations, such as Alcoholics Anonymous, should be appropriately employed. Withdrawal of alcohol usually requires admission to hospital. The severity of symptoms is alleviated by parenteral *chlormethiazole* (Heminevrin). This drug should not be continued for more than a few days because prolonged use may lead to dependency. High potency *vitamin B* should also be given parenterally to prevent a Wernicke–Korsakov syndrome. A *high protein* diet is desirable, provided hepatic encephalopathy is not induced. The management of hepatic failure and encephalopathy is discussed elsewhere.

There is no specific treatment for alcoholic steatosis or cirrhosis. The use of corticosteroids in alcoholic hepatitis is controversial. It should probably be reserved for severe cases. The recommended dose is prednisolone 40 mg daily for approximately 2 weeks.

Prognosis
The prognosis in patients with fatty change alone is excellent, providing consumption of alcohol is controlled. Although steatosis is not a precirrhotic condition, continuance of heavy drinking will lead to hepatitis or cirrhosis in susceptible individuals. At present it is not possible to identify those at particular risk. The majority of patients with hepatitis who continue to drink will go on to cirrhosis. In general, alcoholic cirrhosis has a better prognosis than non-alcoholic cirrhosis. Approximate 5-year survival figures in alcoholic cirrhosis are 60% for abstainers and 40% for persisting drinkers.

Cirrhosis

Categories of cirrhosis – Encephalopathy

The term 'hepatic cirrhosis' should be reserved to describe the combination of diffuse fibrosis and nodular regeneration of the liver parenchyma. It may follow the destruction of normal liver cell architecture from numerous causes. This loss of normal structure may itself lead to further disturbance of hepatic

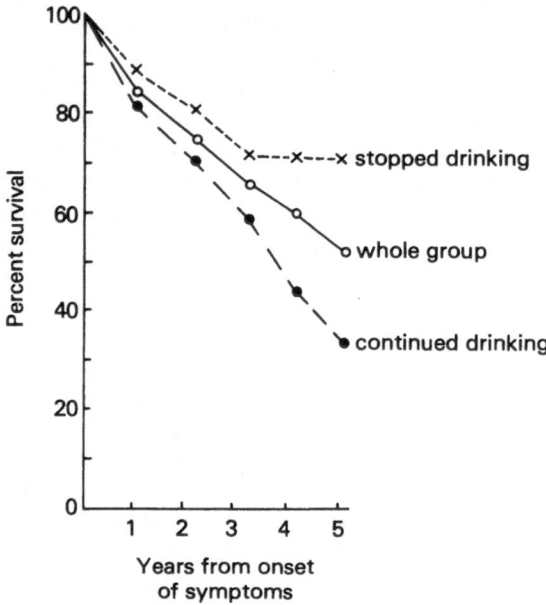

Probability of survival in patients with alcoholic liver disease (based on
Brunt *et al.*, 1974)

Figure 19.2

function, thus causing progression of cirrhosis even after the
initial damaging agent has been removed.

Categories of cirrhosis

There are two major categories based on morphology. *Micronodular* cirrhosis is that in which the regeneration nodules are
small and the whole liver is equally involved. It is most
commonly due to alcohol. *Macronodular* cirrhosis is characterized by much larger regeneration nodules and irregular fibrotic
bands. Some areas of the liver may appear relatively normal.
Viral infection is probably the commonest cause. Some cirrhotic
livers have a mixture of nodule sizes.

The common causes of cirrhosis are:

(1) Type B and type non-A,non-B virus hepatitis
(2) Chronic active hepatitis of any aetiology (p. 178)
(3) Alcohol
(4) Persisting cholestasis (extrahepatic biliary obstruction or
primary biliary cirrhosis).

More rarely it may be the result of longstanding severe cardiac failure. This is most likely to occur when the failure is predominantly right-sided or due to constrictive pericarditis. Deposition of substances such as iron in haemachromatosis, and copper, in Wilson's disease, are other rare causes of cirrhosis. In addition to those cases of known aetiology, there are a significant number in which the cause is unknown. These are labelled 'cryptogenic'. With advancing knowledge and more accurate diagnostic techniques, the proportion in this category has decreased.

Compensated cirrhosis

Many patients with cirrhosis are asymptomatic, the disease being discovered because a medical opinion has been sought for some other reason. It is not uncommon for the pathologist to find cirrhosis at postmortem examination of elderly patients when there has been no suspicion of chronic liver disease during life. In some cases there are vague non-specific symptoms such as lethargy and dyspepsia. Despite the paucity of symptoms, careful examination in such cases will often reveal signs of chronic liver disease. Palmar erythema, spider naevi and mild ankle oedema are usually the most obvious, whilst in the abdomen the spleen and liver are frequently palpable. Splenomegaly is the result of portal venous hypertension which may be present even when hepatocellular function is well preserved. Routine liver function tests may be normal or show only a slight elevation in the serum levels of transaminases or γ-glutamyltranspeptidase. The urine frequently contains an excess of urobilinogen.

Decompensated cirrhosis

With increasing liver cell destruction and structural disruption, the functional capacity is exceeded. This may occur for the first time in patients not suspected of having chronic liver disease because of coincidental infection, an alcoholic binge or gastrointestinal bleeding. The features of decompensated cirrhosis are largely the result of hepatocellular dysfunction. However, they are compounded by the effects of portal venous hypertension which occurs to a variable degree in the majority of cases.

Jaundice   The following features are characteristic of decompensated cirrhosis. Jaundice is usually a sign of severe hepatocyte

193

dysfunction. It is due to a combination of increased haemolysis and decreased conjugation and excretion of bilirubin. Often by the time jaundice has become persistent the previously enlarged liver has shrunk and is no longer palpable.

Encephalo-pathy The mechanism of encephalopathy is not yet understood. It seems likely that bacterial metabolic products formed in the gut are responsible. Detoxification by the diseased liver is impaired and large quantities of portal blood bypass the hepatic sinusoidal system because of the disrupted liver architecture and formation of portosystemic shunts. There is evidence that these metabolites affect brain function by acting as false neurotransmitters which interfere with the normal transmitter substances, dopamine and noradrenalin. Hepatic encephalopathy covers a wide spectrum of neuropsychiatric disturbance. There may be no more than failure of concentration, poor memory and lethargy, but in more serious cases confusion, stupor and coma occur. Characteristic features are a flapping tremor of the outstretched hands and foetor. Pyramidal and extrapyramidal signs are sometimes present.

Bleeding A prolonged prothrombin time due to impaired production of clotting factors is very common and leads to bruising. A reduced platelet count which is mainly the result of hypersplenism causes purpura. Bleeding from varices in the oesophagus and stomach is a very serious complication and is a common cause of death. However, not all gastrointestinal bleeding in cirrhotic patients is variceal. Gastric erosions and peptic ulcer must always be considered.

Ascites and oedema Fluid and sodium retention are common in cirrhosis. The mechanisms are not entirely clear. Increased sodium retention by the kidney partly due to secondary hyperaldosteronism is one factor. Hypoalbuminaemia which results from impaired hepatic production of albumin also encourages oedema formation. Portal hypertension and increased hepatic lymph production are other important factors in the pathogenesis of ascites.

Splenomegaly Enlargement of the spleen in cirrhosis is due to portal venous hypertension. Hypersplenism, by which is meant the increased destruction of platelets and red cells by the enlarged spleen, contributes to the anaemia and thrombocytopenia of cirrhosis.

Endocrine disturbance Impaired glucose tolerance is very common, and approximately one third of patients with cirrhosis have clinical *diabetes*. Testosterone and oestrogen metabolism is abnormal. This leads to *atrophic testes, loss of body hair, gynaecomastia* and *impotence* in male patients.

Bone disease   Both osteomalacia and osteoporosis occur more commonly in cirrhosis than in the general population and result in bone pain and muscle weakness. Osteomalacia is mainly due to poor intake and malabsorption of vitamin D. Failure of hepatorenal conversion of vitamin D to the active compound 1,25-dihydroxy-cholecalciferol is relatively unimportant.

Investigation

Serum bilirubin is frequently raised, although in well compensated cases normal values may be found. The serum *alkaline phosphatase, γ-glutamyltranspeptidase* and *transaminase levels* are usually raised. *Plasma albumin* is decreased and *γ-globulins* are often increased.

Anaemia is common. The film usually shows a normocytic–normochromic picture although macrocytosis is sometimes seen, especially in alcoholic patients. *Reduced white blood cell* counts and *thrombocytopenia* are often present. Impaired synthesis of clotting factors cause a *prolonged prothrombin time.* In contrast to the situation in cholestatic jaundice, the increased prothrombin time is not corrected in cirrhosis by parenteral vitamin K. *Scanning of the liver* after injection of a *radionuclide* shows reduced uptake by the liver but increased radioactivity over the spleen. Cirrhosis also has a typical pattern on *ultrasound scanning.* Both techniques are capable of detecting a coexistent hepatoma.

A *definitive diagnosis of cirrhosis depends upon needle biopsy of the liver.* Histology may suggest the underlying cause, but establishing the aetiology often depends upon clinical features. Special stains are necessary to detect the abnormal deposition of iron in haemochromatosis and copper in Wilson's disease. *Additional blood tests* may also aid the aetiological diagnosis. In primary biliary cirrhosis there is a high titre of mitochondrial antibody, whilst a large proportion of patients with autoimmune chronic active hepatitis have antibodies in the serum to smooth muscle and nucleoprotein. The finding of hepatitis B antigens clearly suggests a viral aetiology. In a patient with cirrhosis who is rapidly deteriorating, a high concentration of serum α-fetoprotein points to a coexistent hepatoma.

Management

Specific   There is no specific therapy for the great majority of patients
therapy   with cirrhosis. There are three exceptions to this. *Haemo-*

chromatosis is treated by repeated venesection to mobilize iron stored in the liver. *Wilson's disease* may be arrested by long term treatment with the chelating agent, penicillamine, which removes copper from the tissues and promotes its excretion in the urine. Prednisolone, with or without azathioprine, is used when there is an associated *chronic active hepatitis.*

Non-specific therapy

In well-compensated cirrhosis no active treatment is required other than (1) abstinence from alcohol and (2) a normal diet.

Fluid and sodium retention

The formation of ascites is a sign of decompensation and results from a combination of hepatocellular failure and portal venous hypertension. It is a serious complication, and when it occurs insidiously the prognosis is particularly poor. In contrast, ascites of sudden onset, which is often precipitated by an alcoholic binge or gastrointestinal haemorrhage, has a better prognosis providing the patient can be adequately supported during the acute phase.

Admission to hospital is usually necessary because the initial treatment requires close monitoring. A small quantity (20–50 ml) of ascitic fluid should be removed for diagnostic purposes. In cirrhotic ascites, the *protein concentration* will be less than 2 g/100 ml. A concentration greater than 3 g/100 ml should raise suspicion of malignancy, infection or hepatic vein thrombosis. *Bloodstaining* usually indicates intra-abdominal cancer, but also occurs in tuberculosis. Low grade infection of ascites is common in cirrhosis and fluid should be cultured routinely. *Cytological examination* in cases of infection will reveal polymorphs, and in cancer malignant cells are frequently present.

Bed rest, together with fluid and sodium restriction, is the mainstay of treatment. The aim is to restrict sodium to 20 mEq/d and fluid to 1 l/d. Adherence to a regime such as this requires the supervision of an enthusiastic dietitian and constant encouragement from medical and nursing staff. Daily weighing, measurement of serum electrolytes and urea and urine output is essential. The aim is to reduce the patient's weight by 500–1000 g per day. If this fails to achieve adequate reduction of ascites within 4 days, a potassium sparing diuretic is given. Spironolactone (Aldactone A) is most commonly used in doses between 50 and 150 mg daily. Amiloride is an alternative. If diuresis is still unsatisfactory, frusemide (Lasix) 40–80 mg or bumetamide (Burinex) 1–2 mg should be started. It may be necessary to increase the dosages to 200 mg or 5 mg respectively. Diuretic therapy may cause hypokalaemia and alkalosis which, in turn, can precipitate encephalopathy. Potassium supplements are frequently required and diuretics may have to be stopped until potassium stores are repleted. A rising blood urea may also indicate overenthusiastic diuretic therapy. This is due to reduction in plasma volume and can be confirmed by the finding of a low central venous pressure. Diuretics should be stopped and fluid volume restored with an infusion of albumin. Many patients with ascites, particularly those resistant to the above regimes, have impaired kidney function due to constriction of intrarenal blood vessels secondary to the liver disease. The mechanism is not clear but is thought to be due to the effect of bacterial endotoxins absorbed from the gut. The prognosis in this group is extremely grave. Treatment consists of fluid, sodium and potassium restriction, but the results are poor.

Recurrence of ascites is very common after discharge from hospital. This is usually due to dietary lapse; persistent encouragement to keep to a 'no added' salt regime (40–60 mEq sodium per day) is therefore necessary. Close monitoring of electrolytes and urea is important in those on maintenance diuretics.

Therapeutic paracentesis of ascites in cirrhosis depletes the body's protein pool. The procedure is potentially dangerous because it may precipitate circulatory failure and encephalopathy. It is now very rarely performed in cirrhosis. In rare cases with resistant ascites, when dietary restriction and diuretic therapy has failed, a LeVeen peritoneo-venous shunt may be implanted. This allows drainage of ascitic fluid from the peritoneum to the internal jugular vein via a subcutaneously implanted synthetic tube.

Encephalo-
pathy
Encephalopathy may be acute or chronic.

There are two main objectives in the management of *acute hepatic encephalopathy* in cirrhosis:

(1) Identification and treatment of the precipitating factor
(2) General measures to alleviate the encephalopathy.

Regarding objective (1), the common precipitating causes of encephalopathy in a previously compensated patient are:

Inappropriate diuretic therapy
Gastrointestinal haemorrhage
An alcoholic binge
Severe diarrhoea and vomiting from any cause
Infections, usually respiratory or urinary tract
Potent analgesics and sedatives
Surgery

197

Constipation
Too much dietary protein
Drainage of large volumes of ascitic fluid.

The general practitioner should be aware of the hazards of using morphine and related analgesics, sedatives and over-enthusiastic diuretic therapy in patients with cirrhosis. The prompt treatment of infections and constipation will often prevent the development of encephalopathy. Nevertheless, it should be stressed that once there is evidence of impending encephalopathy or when the precipitating cause itself requires inpatient treatment, admission should be arranged without delay.

Regarding objective (2), protein should be removed from the diet and 1500–2000 kcal (6.3–8.4 MJ) provided in the form of carbohydrate. If the patient's level of consciousness prevents normal feeding, a nasogastric tube must be used. Only occasionally is the intravenous route required for nutritional purposes. As the encephalopathy improves, a 20 g protein diet in introduced. Protein may then be increased by increments up to a total of 60 g/day. A close watch must be kept on the patient's mental function by the daily performance of simple tests of cerebration. These include copying simple figures, handwriting and trail tests.

Antibiotics *Neomycin*, 1 g 6-hourly, is given by mouth to reduce the gut microflora and thus decrease production of toxic bacterial metabolites. A broad-spectrum antibiotic such as ampicillin is used when bacterial infection is considered to be a possible cause of the encephalopathy.

Lactulose Lactulose (Duphalac, Gatinar) is a sugar which the human intestine is incapable of digesting. It encourages the proliferation of lactose-fermenting organisms at the expense of ammonia and 'toxin'-producing bacteria. It also reduces the pH of the stool, thus decreasing ammonia absorption from the gut. The usual oral dosage in acute encephalopathy is 30 ml q.d.s. It may also be given by enema.

Purgatives and enemas Purgation with magnesium sulphate and colonic lavage with physiological saline both effectively reduce the protein substrate in the bowel.

Blood and intravenous fluids The management of bleeding in patients with cirrhosis has been discussed elsewhere (p. 108). Fluid depletion due to diuretic therapy or diarrhoea and vomiting should be corrected with the appropriate intravenous fluids. Potassium replacement is particularly important. *It should be remembered that although* serum sodium concentrations are often low in cirrhosis, there is seldom a reduction of total body sodium. This is especially true in patients with ascites and infusions with sodium-containing fluids must be avoided in such cases.

Chronic encephalopathy

The neuropsychiatric features of chronic hepatic encephalopathy may be alleviated by restriction of dietary protein and long term use of lactulose or neomycin. Because some types of hepatic encephalopathy resemble Parkinsonism in which brain dopamine is depleted, *levodopa* has been used. Unfortunately, it has no lasting effect. *Bromocriptine*, a dopamine agonist, has also been tried, but further studies are required before it can be recommended for routine use. In resistant cases, *colectomy* or *colonic exclusion* operations are sometimes employed as a means of reducing bacterial 'toxin' production. *Transplantation* of a donor liver has been of limited success in a few cases.

Osteomalacia

The bone pain of osteomalacia can be successfully treated with intramuscular vitamin D, 100 000–150 000 units weekly. The serum calcium and bone alkaline phosphatase levels must be monitored and a suitable maintenance dose found by trial in each patient.

Loss of libido and impotence

The problem of reduced libido and impotence usually proves resistant to treatment. Nevertheless, testosterone orally or as a long acting intramuscular injection is worth trying.

Points to stress

Deterioration of mental function in a patient with cirrhosis

This is most commonly due to:
- Inappropriate use of analgesics, sedatives and diuretics
- Constipation
- Infection
- Gastrointestinal haemorrhage.

Hepatic ascites

- Hepatic ascites is controlled by sodium and fluid restriction and diuretics.
- Drainage of large volumes is dangerous.

20 Common pancreatic diseases

Acute pancreatitis – Chronic pancreatitis

Acute pancreatitis

There are two major clinical subgroups of acute pancreatitis:

(1) Acute pancreatitis refers to a single episode of inflammation of the pancreatic gland.
(2) Relapsing acute pancreatitis which is characterized by recurrent attacks of inflammation.

In both types the gland returns to normal within a few weeks of the acute attack.

Aetiology and pathogenesis

Cholelithiasis In the British Isles cholelithiasis appears to be an important causative factor in more than 50 per cent of cases. The next most common identifiable cause of acute exacerbations of

Alcohol abuse pancreatitis is *alcohol abuse*. There is considerable discussion about whether alcohol-induced pancreatitis fulfills the strict classification of acute pancreatitis because many authorities believe that by the time 'acute alcoholic pancreatitis' presents there are already permanent structural and functional changes within the gland. In the majority of remaining cases there is *no identifiable cause*. In a small number *viruses* have been implicated, the most common being mumps, Coxsackie B and glandular fever. An increasing number of *drugs* have been reported as possible causes of acute pancreatitis. The evidence is strongest against corticosteroids, thiazide diuretics, pheno-

201

thiazines and the contraceptive pill. *Surgery to the abdomen particularly on the stomach and biliary system may be complicated by postoperative pancreatitis. It should also be borne in mind that an episode of pancreatitis may be the first presentation of pancreatic cancer. Hyperlipidaemia, hypercalcaemia* and a *penetrating duodenal ulcer* are rare identifiable causes. Other situations in which pancreatitis occurs more often than can be explained by chance are: pregnancy, renal and hepatic failure, hypothermia and connective tissue disease.

No matter what initiates the inflammation, much of the damage to the gland is brought about by autodigestion of tissue by enzymes released from pancreatic cells. The pathological features vary from the relatively mild oedematous pancreatitis to the very severe haemorrhagic pancreatitis in which there may be total necrosis of the gland.

Symptoms and signs

For practical purposes most cases can be divided into either mild acute pancreatitis or severe fulminant pancreatitis. The former is usually accompanied by the oedematous type of pathology and the latter by haemorrhagic necrotizing changes.

Mild pancreatitis

Mild pancreatitis – Upper abdominal pain which frequently radiates to the back is the characteristic presentation. It is accompanied by nausea and vomiting. The features of shock are absent or minimal and on examination of the abdomen the only abnormality is moderate guarding. Pain usually lasts for no more than a few days and prognosis is good.

Fulminant pancreatitis

Severe fulminant pancreatitis – In this group abdominal pain is intense and accompanied by persistent vomiting. Signs of peritonism are present and paralytic ileus is very common. This type of pancreatitis is frequently accompanied by pleural effusions, basal atelectasis, bruising in the flanks or around the umbilicus and pseudocyst or abscess.

Systemic disturbance is always present and varies from a mild pyrexia with leucocytosis to profound shock with oliguria, coma and 'stress' ulceration of the upper alimentary tract.

Other common metabolic disturbances are hypocalcaemia, hyperglycaemia, hyperlipidaemia and disseminated intravascular coagulation.

Patients in whom pain and systemic disturbance persists for more than a week should be suspected of having a *pseudocyst* or *abscess*.

Common pancreatic diseases

Diagnosis

Blood tests   The most useful test in confirming the diagnosis is the *serum amylase concentration*. Very high levels (over 1000 international units per litre) are strongly indicative of acute pancreatitis. Lower levels (between 300 and 1000 international units per litre) are found in pancreatitis but may also occur in other acute intrabdominal disease of which gall bladder disease, perforated peptic ulcer, hepatitis and gut ischaemia are the most common. *However, patients with mild pancreatitis may have normal levels of serum amylase and paradoxically in some cases of fulminant disease concentrations in the serum are equivocal.* The level of serum amylase does not therefore accurately reflect the severity of disease. Serial estimations are valuable. Levels usually fall within a few days but persistent elevation strongly suggests a pseudocyst.

Serum lipase estimation is not commonly performed. This test may be of use if the patient who presents late or when the diagnosis of pancreatitis was not initially considered, because levels rise later than those of amylase and remain high for a longer period. Modest elevations of serum bilirubin, alkaline phosphatase and transaminases are very common but do not necessarily indicate that acute pancreatitis is secondary to gallstones.

Radiology   An X-ray film of the abdomen may reveal a dilated sentinel loop of small bowel high in the abdomen, or gallstones.

Ultrasound   Ultrasonography has become the investigation of choice to confirm inflammatory changes or to detect the presence of a pseudocyst or abscess.

Treatment

The aims of treatment are to:

- reduce inflammation
- relieve pain
- prevent and treat complications.

Reduction of inflammation

(a) There is a good theoretical basis for 'resting' the pancreas by stopping all oral food and liquid and providing *nutrition by the parenteral route.*

(b) *Aspiration of gastric contents* reduces stimulation of the pancreas and risk of vomiting.

(c) Although *anticholinergic drugs* reduce pancreatic

203

secretion there is no sound evidence that they reduce morbidity or mortality.

(d) Neither *antacids or cimetidine* have been found useful in the management of acute pancreatitis, despite the reduction of pancreatic secretion that should result from increasing the pH of gastric contents.

(e) *Glucagon* inhibits pancreatic exocrine function, but controlled trials have not shown any clinical advantages from its use.

(f) *Calcitonin* inhibits pancreatic secretion and there is early evidence that it may reduce both severity and duration of acute pancreatitis.

(g) *Proteinase inhibitors* – Because much of the damage to the pancreas results from autodigestion, enzyme inhibition would seem to be a logical treatment. However, neither aprotinin (Trasylol) or epsilon aminocaproic acid have been found of use in the clinical situation.

(h) *Peritoneal dialysis*, by removing large quantities of damaging pancreatic enzymes and inflammation-inducing kinins and toxins, may have a part to play, but full clinical trials are awaited.

Pain relief — Pentazocine (Fortral) in adequate doses is effective in acute pancreatitis and has the advantage over morphine derivatives and pethidine that it does not cause contraction of the sphincter of Oddi. However, when pain is severe this latter group of drugs may be necessary. Epidural blockade with local anaesthesia is an alternative when parenteral analgesia fails.

Prevention of complications — *Shock.* The prevention of shock is dependent upon close monitoring and early correction of metabolic and haemodynamic disturbances. For this reason all but the mildest cases should be admitted to an intensive care unit.

Respiratory impairment may be eased by increasing the concentration of oxygen inspired but when the shock lung syndrome threatens positive end expiratory pressure should be used.

Renal failure that does not respond to adequate intravenous fluid replacement may require correction by peritoneal or haemodialysis.

Surgery — Despite the use of the diagnostic tests previously discussed, *laparotomy* may be necessary to confirm the diagnosis and exclude other causes of the acute abdomen. Most authorities believe that removal of gallstones should be delayed until the acute inflammation has settled.

Many pseudocysts resolve spontaneously over a period of

several weeks but some eventually require drainage. An abscess or infected cyst should be drained.

Prognosis   Mortality from acute pancreatitis is approximately 20 per cent. Poor prognosis is associated with old age, shock, disseminated intravascular coagulation, a rising blood urea and hypocalcaemia. In those who recover, pancreatic function is normal. Investigation for the known predisposing causes should be undertaken as soon as possible.

Chronic pancreatitis

Chronic pancreatitis can be defined as a chronic inflammatory condition of the pancreas which has led to permanent dysfunction. Acute inflammatory exacerbations may be superimposed and this is termed '*chronic relapsing pancreatitis*'.

Aetiology and   The commonest known causes in the United Kingdom are
pathogenesis   alcohol abuse and probably cholelithiasis. It may also occur rarely after repeated episodes of acute pancreatitis associated with hyperparathyroidism and hyperlipidaemia. Cystic fibrosis in children and adolescents and haemochromatosis in adults also lead to chronic pancreatic insufficiency. When due to alcohol, the inflammatory process is initiated by plugs of proteinaceous matter which obstruct the ducts. This eventually leads to atrophy of the glandular acini, cyst formation, fibrosis and calcification.

Symptoms and   *Upper abdominal pain* radiating to the back is the predom-
signs   inant presenting symptom. The usual description is a 'deep, boring ache' or 'cramp'. Severity varies, but some attacks may necessitate admission to hospital for adequate analgesic treatment. Acute pain may last for several days and is then often followed by a continuing dull ache for several weeks. Alcohol is a common precipitating or exacerbating factor. Leaning forward or lying prone may give relief. About 10% of all cases have no pain and present with other clinical features. *Anorexia* and *loss of weight* are common. In approximately 40%, *malabsorption* with *steatorrhoea* contribute to weight loss and malnutrition. Two thirds have a diabetic glucose tolerance test and in one third there is clinical *diabetes*. On examination, *tenderness* in the epigastrium will be present during the acute phase. A *pseudocyst* may also be palpable. Obstructive *jaundice* is often seen due to oedema or fibrosis around the common bile duct.

Diagnosis   The serum or urinary amylase levels may be raised during acute exacerbations, but normal levels do not exclude the

205

diagnosis. Between acute episodes, enzyme levels are almost invariably normal. A persistently elevated level is found when a pseudocyst or abscess has formed. Steatorrhoea can be confirmed by *faecal fat estimation* (p. 88). *Pancreatic exocrine dysfunction*, assessed by the pancreozymin–secretin or Lundh tests, is the usual means of confirming the diagnosis (p. 89). An *X-ray of the abdomen* reveals calcification in the gland in 30% of cases. *Endoscopic retrograde pancreatography* (p. 89) is now commonly employed to demonstrate the abnormal duct system in chronic pancreatitis. *Grey scale ultrasound and computerized axial tomography* are useful in the diagnosis of acute inflammation, pseudocysts and abscess of the pancreas. It may be necessary to resort to *laparotomy* in some cases.

Management   The treatment of acute attacks has been discussed (p. 203). Persisting pain can often be relieved by simple analgesics such as aspirin or paracetamol, but more potent drugs are sometimes needed. Because of the chronic nature of the disease, addictive compounds should be avoided whenever possible. There must be total abstinence from alcohol. A cholecystectomy should be performed when gallstones are present. Hyperparathyroidism and hyperlipidaemia are treated appropriately.

Malabsorption is reduced by pancreatic supplements taken at mealtimes (Pancrex, Nutrizyme). Antacids and cimetidine are also of value because they reduce gastric acid and, therefore, lessen the destruction of both endogenous and exogenous pancreatic enzymes. Fat restriction may be necessary if clinical steatorrhoea remains a problem. Codeine phosphate and loperamide are useful for the symptomatic relief of diarrhoea.

Diabetes usually requires insulin, although the occasional patient can be managed on oral hypoglycaemic drugs. These measures are successful in approximately 50% of patients, particularly if there is total abstinence from alcohol.

If pain continues, surgery should be considered. This may consist of either *drainage procedures* to bypass obstructed ducts or *resection* of diseased gland. *Blocking the coeliac ganglion* is an alternative measure when surgery is contraindicated.

Further reading

Oesophageal Disease
> Topics in Gastroenterology 4, ed. Truelove & Ritchie (Oxford: Blackwell Scientific Publications)
> Clinics in Gastroenterology vol. 5, no. 1, Disorders of Oesophageal Motility, ed. Atkinson (New York: W. B. Saunders)

Peptic Ulcer
> Topics in Gastroenterology 1, ed. Truelove & Jewell (Oxford: Blackwell Scientific Publications)
> Topics in Gastroenterology 7, ed. Truelove & Willoughby (Oxford: Blackwell Scientific Publications)
> Topics in Gastroenterology 6, ed. Truelove & Heyworth (Oxford: Blackwell Scientific Publications)

Gastrointestinal Haemorrhage
> Clinics in Gastroenterology vol. 10, no. 1, Gastrointestinal Emergencies, ed. Torsoli (New York: W. B. Saunders)
> Topics in Gastroenterology 3, ed. Truelove & Goodman (Oxford: Blackwell Scientific Publications)

Irritable Bowel Syndrome
> Topics in Gastroenterology 1, ed. Truelove & Jewell (Oxford: Blackwell Scientific Publications)
> Clinics in Gastroenterology vol. 6, no. 3, The G. I. Tract in Stress and Psychological Disorder, ed. Almy & Fielding (New York: W. B. Saunders)

Inflammatory Bowel Disease
> Topics in Gastroenterology, 1, ed. Truelove & Jewell (Oxford: Blackwell Scientific Publications)
> Topics in Gastroenterology, 8, ed. Truelove & Kennedy (Oxford: Blackwell Scientific Publications)

Coeliac Disease
> Topics in Gastroenterology, 4, ed. Truelove & Ritchie (Oxford: Blackwell Scientific Publications)
> Immunology of the G. I. Tract, ed. Asquith (Edinburgh: Churchill Livingstone)

Liver & Biliary System – General
> Liver & Biliary Disease, ed. Wright, Alberti, Karvan & Millward-Sailler (New York: W. B. Saunders)
> Diseases of Liver & Biliary System, Sherlock (Oxford: Blackwell Scientific Publications)

Hepatitis
> Topics in Gastroenterology, 3, ed. Truelove & Goodman (Oxford: Blackwell Scientific Publications)
> Topics in Gastroenterology, 4, ed. Truelove & Ritchie (Oxford: Blackwell Scientific Publications)
> Topics in Gastroenterology, 6, ed. Truelove & Heyworth (Oxford: Blackwell Scientific Publications)

Drugs and the Liver
> Topics in Gastroenterology, 5, ed. Truelove & Lee (Oxford: Blackwell Scientific Publications)

Gastrointestinal Cancer
> Cancer of the G. I. Tract. Clinics in Gastroenterology vol. 5, no. 3, ed. Sherlock & Zamcheck (New York: W. B. Saunders)

Gastroenteritis
> Infections of the G. I. Tract. Clinics in Gastroenterology, ed. Lambert (New York: W. B. Saunders)

The Acute Abdomen
> Gastrointestinal Emergencies. Clinics in Gastroenterology, ed. Torsoli (New York: W. B. Saunders)

Index